THE TRUTH ABOUT STRESS MANAGEMENT

ROBERT N. GOLDEN, M.D.
University of Wisconsin–Madison
General Editor

FRED L. PETERSON, PH.D.
University of Texas–Austin
General Editor

THOMAS STREISSGUTH
Principal Author

HEATH DINGWELL, PH.D.
Contributing Author

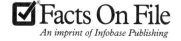
Facts On File
An imprint of Infobase Publishing

Facts On File, Inc.
An imprint of Infobase Publishing
132 West 31st Street
New York NY 10001

Library of Congress Cataloging-in-Publication Data

Streissguth, Thomas, 1958–
    The truth about stress management / Thomas Streissguth. – 1st ed.
      p. cm.
    Includes bibliographical references and index.
    ISBN-13: 978-0-8160-7647-5 (hardcover : alk. paper)
      10: 0-8160-7647-2 (hardcover : alk. paper) 1. Stress management for teenagers—Juvenile literature. I. Title.
      BF724.3.S86S77 2011
      155.5'18–dc22

                                                                    2010020750

Facts On File books are available at special discounts when purchased in bulk quantities for businesses, associations, institutions, or sales promotions. Please call our Special Sales Department in New York at (212) 967-8800 or (800) 322-8755.

You can find Facts On File on the World Wide Web at http://www.factsonfile.com.

Text design by David Strelecky
Composition by Mary Susan Ryan-Flynn
Cover printed by Art Print, Taylor, Pa.
Book printed and bound by Maple Press, York, Pa.
Date printed: March 2011

Printed in the United States of America

10 9 8 7 6 5 4 3 2 1

This book is printed on acid-free paper.

CONTENTS

LIST OF ILLUSTRATIONS AND TABLES

PREFACE

The Truth About series—updated and expanded to include 20 volumes—seeks to identify the most pressing health issues and social challenges confronting our nation's youth. Adolescence is the period between the onset of puberty and the attainment of adult roles and responsibilities. Adolescence is also a time of storm, stress, and risk-taking for many young people. During adolescence, a person's health is influenced by biological, psychological, and social factors, all of which interact with one's environment—family, peers, school, and community. It is a time when teenagers experience profound changes.

With the latest available statistics and new insights that have emerged from ongoing research, the Truth About series seeks to help young people build a foundation of information as they face some of the challenges that will affect their health and well-being. These challenges include high-risk behaviors, such as alcohol, tobacco, and other drug use; sexual behaviors that can lead to adolescent pregnancy and sexually transmitted diseases (STDs), such as HIV/AIDS; mental health concerns, such as depression and suicide; learning disorders and disabilities, which are often associated with failure at school and dropping out of school; serious family problems, including domestic violence and abuse; and lifestyle choices, which can increase adolescents' risk for noncommunicable diseases, such as diabetes and cardiovascular disease.

Broader underlying factors also influence adolescent health. These include socioeconomic circumstances, such as poverty, available health care, and the political and social situations in which young people live. Although these factors can negatively affect adolescent health and well-being, as well as school performance, many of these negative health outcomes are preventable with the proper knowledge and information.

With prevention in mind, the writers and editors of each topical volume in the Truth About series have tried to provide cutting-edge information that is supported by research and scientific evidence. Vital facts are presented that inform youth about the challenges experienced during adolescence, while special features seek to dispel common myths and misconceptions. Some of the main topics explored include abuse, alcohol, death and dying, divorce, drugs, eating disorders, family life, fear and depression, rape, sexual behavior and unplanned pregnancy, smoking, and violence. All volumes discuss risk-taking behaviors and their consequences, healthy choices, prevention, available treatments, and where to get help.

In this new edition of the series, we also have added eight new titles in areas of increasing significance to today's youth. ADHD, or attention-deficit/hyperactivity disorder, and learning disorders are diagnosed with increasing frequency, and many students have observed or know of classmates receiving treatment for these conditions, even if they have not themselves received this diagnosis. Gambling is gaining currency in our culture, as casinos open and expand in many parts of the country, and the Internet offers easy access for this addictive behavior. Another consequence of our increasingly "online" society, unfortunately, is the presence of online predators. Environmental hazards represent yet another danger, and it is important to provide unbiased information about this topic to our youth. Suicide, which for many years has been a "silent epidemic," is now gaining recognition as a major public health problem throughout the life span, including the teenage and young adult years. We now also offer an overview of illness and disease in a volume that includes the major conditions of particular interest and concern to youth. In addition to illness, however, it is essential to emphasize health and its promotion, and this is especially apparent in the volumes on physical fitness and stress management.

It is our intent that each book serve as an accessible, authoritative resource to which young people can turn for accurate and meaningful answers to their specific questions. The series can help them research particular problems and provide an up-to-date evidence base. It is also designed with parents, teachers, and counselors in mind so that they have a reliable resource that they can share with youth who seek their guidance.

Finally, we have tried to provide unbiased facts rather than subjective opinions. Our goal is to help elevate the health of the public with an emphasis on its most precious component—our youth. As young people face the challenges of an increasingly complex world, we as educators want them to be armed with the most powerful weapon available—knowledge.

Robert N. Golden, M.D.
Fred L. Peterson, Ph.D.
General Editors

HOW TO
USE THIS BOOK

NOTE TO STUDENTS

Knowledge is power. By possessing knowledge you have the ability to make decisions, ask follow-up questions, and know where to go to obtain more information. In the world of health, that is power! That is the purpose of this book—to provide you the power you need to obtain unbiased, accurate information and *The Truth About Stress Management.*

Topics in each volume of the Truth About are arranged in alphabetical order, from A to Z. Each of these entries defines its topic and explains in detail the particular issue. At the end of most entries are cross-references to related topics. A list of all topics by letter can be found in the table of contents or at the back of the book in the index.

How have these books been compiled? First, the publisher worked with me to identify some of the country's leading authorities on key issues in health education. These individuals were asked to identify some of the major concerns that young people have about such topics. The writers read the literature, spoke with health experts, and incorporated their own life and professional experiences to pull together the most up-to-date information on health issues, particularly those of interest to adolescents and of concern in Healthy People 2010.

Throughout the alphabetical entries, the reader will find sidebars that separate Fact from Fiction. There are Question-and-Answer boxes that attempt to address the most common questions that youth ask about sensitive topics. In addition, readers will find a special feature called "Teens Speak"—case studies of teens with personal stories related to the topic in hand.

This may be one of the most important books you will ever read. Please share it with your friends, families, teachers, and classmates. Remember, you possess the power to control your future. One way to affect your course is through the acquisition of knowledge. Good luck and keep healthy.

NOTE TO LIBRARIANS

This book, along with the rest of the series the Truth About, serves as a wonderful resource for young researchers. It contains a variety of facts, case studies, and further readings that the reader can use to help answer questions, formulate new questions, or determine where to go to find more information. Even though the topics may be considered delicate by some, don't be afraid to ask patrons if they have questions. Feel free to direct them to the appropriate sources, but do not press them if you encounter reluctance. The best we can do as educators is to let young people know that we are there when they need us.

STRESS IS NOT NECESSARILY BAD

Stress is a part of life. Chances are likely that as you read this book, you are experiencing stress. According to the Nemours Foundation, one of the country's leading pediatric health-care systems, stress is a feeling that is created when we react to particular events. Stress itself is neither good nor bad; it is a physical reaction to events that occur in our lives.

The human body is a complex system designed to navigate and survive the world. Our senses—taste, sound, smell, and sight—help guide us. As we experience and learn about the world, we become even better prepared to navigate life. Collectively, our senses, intuition, and experience help us survive and, with luck, thrive. However, even when we are not "fighting" to survive, our bodies are always working to manage our reactions.

TYPES OF STRESS

There are several different types of stress: **eustress, distress, acute stress, chronic stress, hyperstress,** and **hypostress.**

Eu- comes from Greek and means "well" or "good." Eustress refers to positive stress. This type of stress is said to enhance the body's ability to function. Positive events in life, such as playing sports or spending time with friends, can be viewed as eustress.

Distress, the opposite of eustress, refers to negative stress. Distress can cause anxiety, **depression,** suffering, and so forth. Getting into fights with friends, failing a test, breaking up with a boyfriend or girlfriend, and the death of a loved one are examples of distress.

Acute and chronic stress are two types of distress. Acute stress comes and goes in a short period of time. Chronic stress lasts longer; it can continue for days, weeks, months, or even years. Hyperstress refers to a person's experiencing too much stress. Hypostress is the state of being bored and not experiencing enough stress in life.

STRESS AND STUDENTS

The American College Health Association, which collects data on college students, found some interesting information related to stress. The organization's survey, the National College Health Assessment, is administered in the fall and spring semesters of each year. In fall 2008, results indicated that stress was the number one impediment to academic performance. Slightly more than 27 percent of students indicated that stress is an impediment. The second most common problem among college students was difficulty with sleep, coming in at 19.2 percent. Anxiety was the third most common problem at 18.2 percent.

MANAGING STRESS

Because stress is an unavoidable part of life, people need to find ways to deal with it, and that is why stress management is important. Properly dealing with stress is more important than being subjected to stress. People only have so much control over what happens to them. However, they have complete control over how they react to situations.

Unfortunately, many people feel there is not much they can do to deal with stress. Although it may be difficult to deal with specific circumstances, people can do many things to reduce the physical and psychological toll of these events.

Exercise is one of the best ways to deal with stress in a healthy manner. Exercise has been shown to reduce blood pressure and improve psychological functioning. In particular, exercise can help to improve the symptoms of depression and anxiety.

Meditation and Stress

Many experts recommend meditation as one of the best ways to handle stress. This "time-honored" method not only reduces stress but also can make positive changes in life. According to the National Center for Complementary and Alternative Medicine, a branch of the National Institutes of Health, meditation "refers to a variety of techniques or practices intended to focus or control attention." Meditation involves going into a deep state of relaxation. Relaxing the body helps calm the mind. There are probably times where your thoughts are going a "million miles a minute" because of stress. By using meditation, people learn to calm the mind. In turn, people can take better control of their reactions to stress.

Medication and Stress

Sometimes medications are needed and can enable people to deal with stress in their lives. Antidepressants, for example, the class of medications used to help control anxiety and depressive disorders, are used to help people function better. With overwhelming stress, many stressors may occur at once—losing a job, having a relative die, experiencing severe financial difficulties, and so forth. Extreme stress can overwhelm the mind and body. In these cases, doctors often prescribe medications either temporarily or for long-term use. Some people have chemical imbalances in the brain that cause them to be predisposed to anxiety or depressive disorders. For those individuals, handling stress can be more difficult simply because of these chemical imbalances.

With the use of some antidepressants, there may be an increased risk of suicidal thoughts or attempts at suicide. Pharmaceutical companies are required to inform people of these potential risks. However, this concern is controversial. While some data indicated people on antidepressants were at an increased risk of suicidal thoughts or behavior, other studies have indicated that medications play no such role. As with any prescription medication, it is important to follow a doctor's directions when taking antidepressants.

SOURCES OF STRESS

Stress is found in all aspects of life. Family, school, work, and friends are all sources of stress. For example, the authors of a 2009 article in *Social Science and Medicine* reviewed evidence that workplace status is related to heart disease. In particular, they found that the higher a person's job status is, the lower his or her risk of heart disease and hypertension. The lower one's job status, the more likely a person is to suffer from these conditions. In other words, job status is inversely related to heart disease. In fact, according to the authors of a 2008 article in the *European Heart Journal,* approximately one-third of coronary heart disease can be attributed to stress at work.

CONSEQUENCES OF STRESS

Stress takes a toll on the body, especially for people who lack the skills necessary to constructively deal with the stress.

The authors of a 2007 article in *Physiological Reviews* discuss the "weathering hypothesis." This hypothesis argues that stress accelerates the aging process. Looking at the president of the United States, for example, provides an excellent picture of the toll stress takes on the body. Conduct an Internet search for photos of President Bill Clinton, or George W. Bush, when he was first elected and then at the end of his term. For President Obama, compare a photo when he was elected to what he looks like even a year into his first term. One thing you will immediately notice is hair color. Their hair turned white or gray quickly. Hair color can change as a result of the hormones the body produces during stressful periods. Presidents are subjected to years of chronic stress.

One of the hormones involved in the body's response to stress is called **cortisol.** This hormone is vital to the stress response, as it helps the body prepare to react. However, cortisol is not intended to remain at an elevated level in the body for long periods of time. If this happens, it can suppress the body's immune system, cause problems with the cardiovascular system, damage muscles, harm the thyroid, and cause other unwanted consequences.

Authors of a 2009 article in *Revisão Review* found that people who react more strongly to stress have a higher increase in their blood pressure. They were 21 percent more likely to have this increase compared to those who do not respond with a great deal of emotional intensity. People who express their emotions, both positive and negative, in a healthy manner experience a smaller increase in blood pressure. In a study published in a 2009 issue of the *Journal of Cross-Cultural Psychology,* researchers reported this finding. However, the authors noted that a person's culture also influences this reaction.

Psychological stress also has an effect on cardiovascular disease. The author of an article in a 2008 issue of the *Journal of the American College of Cardiology* reviewed evidence that stress is related to sudden death, heart function abnormalities, tissue death in the heart, and insufficient blood supply to the heart.

POST-TRAUMATIC STRESS DISORDER

One possible reaction to severe stress is **post-traumatic stress disorder (PTSD).** According to the U.S. Department of Veterans Affairs,

PTSD is "an anxiety disorder that can occur after you have been through a traumatic event." Trauma involves scary events when your life or the lives of others are in danger. Car accidents, fights, disasters such as earthquakes or tornadoes, witnessing someone die, and combat situations are some types of traumatic events. The emotions associated with these events can trigger changes in the brain that lead to PTSD. Symptoms of the disorder include: reliving the event, avoiding similar situations, feeling numb, and always being alert or jittery (hyperarousal).

The Department of Veterans Affairs estimates that 8 percent of men and 20 percent of women will develop PTSD after a traumatic event. This translates into slightly more than 5 million people dealing with PTSD in any given year. Members of the military who go to war are especially prone to developing PTSD. It is estimated that 12 to 20 percent of the 2003 Iraq War veterans suffer from PTSD. On a wider scale, approximately 30 percent of Vietnam War veterans are believed to have suffered from PTSD.

Although the sources of stress cannot be avoided in life, managing reactions to stress and honing abilities to constructively deal with difficult situations is an essential life skill.

RISKY BUSINESS SELF-TESTS: TRUE OR FALSE

The following tests are designed to let you find out more about the stressors in your life and how well you cope with them. The first test asks about sources of stress in your life. The second asks about unhealthy stress management tactics. The last asks you to examine healthier ways to deal with stress. Record your answers on a separate sheet of paper.

Sources of stress

Answer "true" or "false" to each of the following questions.

_____ I expect a lot from myself.

_____ My parents have high expectations of me.

_____ I struggle to do well in school.

_____ I do not have many friends.

_____ I often feel nervous.

_____ I do not get along with my parents.

_____ Other people my age do not understand me.

_____ Other kids pick on me.

_____ I have a lot of personal problems.

_____ I recently broke up with my boy- or girlfriend.

The more items that are true, the more stress you have in your life.

Unhealthy stress management techniques
Answer "true" or "false" to each of these questions.

_____ I smoke when stressed.

_____ I drink alcohol to forget my problems.

_____ I use drugs to get away from my problems.

_____ I keep my emotions bottled up.

_____ I often stew over what other people have done to me.

_____ There is no one I can talk to about my problems.

_____ I often get into fights with people who cause me problems.

_____ I am often angry.

_____ There is nothing I can do to improve the problems in my life.

_____ I eat unhealthy food to deal with my problems.

The more items that are true, the more problems you have dealing properly with stress.

Healthy stress management techniques
Answer "true" or "false" to each of the following questions.

_____ I exercise to relieve stress.

_____ I talk to other people about the problems in my life.

_____ I look for acceptable solutions to problems in my life.

_____ I think before I speak.

_____ I use meditation or visualization techniques to relax.

_____ I use deep breathing to help calm down.

_____ When I am angry, I walk away from a problem to cool off.

_____ I do not let little problems get to me.

_____ I devote at least 15 minutes a day to just relaxing.

_____ I try to stay positive when problems arise.

The more items that are true, the better you handle the stressors in your life.

A-TO-Z ENTRIES

■ ANNIVERSARY REACTIONS

Physical and psychological reactions to prior traumatic events. Anniversary reactions can occur on a yearly basis after a traumatic event. The trigger may be the death of a relative or friend, or a wide-scale disaster. People who experience anniversary reactions may become irritable, depressed, angry, and sick, among other symptoms. Little is known about why some people experience these reactions. Recent research now links anniversary reactions to post-traumatic stress disorder.

SYMPTOMS AND RESEARCH

Anniversary reactions can occur in response to prior traumatic events, often on a yearly basis, around the date on which the trauma had occurred. Some of the common psychological symptoms include grieving, frustration, anger, sadness, guilt, irritability, sleeplessness, and avoidance. People may also experience physical symptoms, such as catching a cold or becoming severely sick.

The National Center for Post-Traumatic Stress Disorder states that avoidance, arousal, and re-experiencing symptoms can occur on the anniversary of a traumatic event. Avoidance symptoms involve trying to avoid anything that may cause a person to relive the disturbing event. That may involve steering clear of people or places for a period of time.

Arousal symptoms refer to both physical and emotional arousal. These symptoms can include irritability, fear, anxiety, headaches, general nervousness, and so on. The Center for PTSD reports that re-experiencing the event is in fact the most common anniversary reaction.

Unlike other topics of stress management, there has not been much research on this phenomenon. Interestingly, Sigmund Freud first discussed this concept back in 1895. During the early and mid-1900s, some research was also done on the topic, followed up in the 1970s and 1980s. However, only occasional research on anniversary reactions has appeared since. Work from 1990 through the present has focused on anniversary reactions in which the person suffered from post-traumatic stress disorder. A person does not have to suffer from PTSD, however, in order to experience an anniversary reaction.

According to the authors of a 1999 paper in the *Journal of Contemporary Psychotherapy,* when children are traumatized, they often feel guilty about the traumatic event. It is believed that if a parent dies, for example, guilty feelings arise in a child because of parent-child conflicts that had never been resolved. As the authors note, children and adolescents often do not receive the guidance they need to properly cope with anniversary reactions.

CAUSES OF ANNIVERSARY REACTIONS

Because little is known about why people experience anniversary reactions, given the lack of research on the topic, it is difficult to explain them. The most common explanation states that anniversary reactions are the result of incomplete mourning. A 1992 article in the *Clinical Social Work Journal* states this position best: An anniversary reaction is "a pathological consequence of inadequately mourning a traumatic loss." As a result, a person goes through another period of mourning on the anniversary of a traumatic event. The physical and psychological symptoms a person experiences are part of this mourning process.

TEENS SPEAK

I Have to Deal With My Dad's Death Every Year

My dad died when I was eight. Losing him was the hardest thing I'd experienced. Even with counseling I was upset for most of the following year. I had been making progress, but as the first year of his death approached, I became sick. I became more depressed and was angry at the world again. The counselor told me this was normal and I would get better as time went on. I did, but every year around the time of his death I grew sad again. It's not as bad as it used to be, but it will probably always be a hard time for me.

With more studies, research will offer more answers to why anniversary reactions occur. For now, the research, including the studies discussed in this section, essentially examine the prevalence of these reactions and common symptoms that accompany them.

EVIDENCE OF ANNIVERSARY REACTIONS

There are several studies that examine evidence of anniversary reactions. The authors of a 2008 study in the *Journal of Traumatic*

Stress examined anniversary reactions of mental health workers who responded to the 9/11 terrorist attacks. These were the people who helped counsel rescue workers trying to find survivors of the terrorist attacks. On the one-year anniversary, many of the mental health workers were found to have an increasingly negative mood and could not function properly. There was an increase in PTSD symptoms.

An interesting study appeared in a 2007 issue of the *Journal of Nervous and Mental Disease*. The authors wanted to know if watching anniversary coverage of the 9/11 attacks caused people to show signs of post-traumatic stress disorder. Residents of the New York City metropolitan area were studied. The authors found that people who watched more than 12 hours of anniversary coverage were 3.34 times more likely than those watching fewer than four hours to indicate symptoms of PTSD. People who did not experience any symptoms of PTSD right after the attacks were given a diagnosis of new-onset probable PTSD if they watched more than 12 hours of anniversary coverage. This means that people show enough symptoms to probably have PTSD; however, a definitive diagnosis could not be made. "New-onset" indicates the probable PTSD is due to recent events—in this case, due to watching extended coverage of the 9/11 anniversary.

Fact Or Fiction?

Anniversary reactions occur only when a person is aware of the anniversary.

The Facts: People do not have to be aware of an anniversary to experience negative reactions. Although the person may not consciously remember the anniversary, a person can remember at the subconscious level and start experiencing distressing symptoms.

One group that has been repeatedly studied is Persian Gulf war veterans. The authors of a 1998 article in the *Journal of Traumatic Stress* examined anniversary reactions in veterans two years after the 1991 gulf war ended. The authors found that anniversary reactions occurred in combat veterans. Specifically, those who experienced anniversary reactions showed significantly higher levels of hostility, depression, and obsessive-compulsive behavior. They also scored higher on measures of post-traumatic stress disorder. In fact, the authors discovered that 100 percent of veterans who were diagnosed with PTSD experienced anniversary reactions. By comparison, only 20 percent of veterans without PTSD experienced these reactions.

Several authors of the first study conducted a follow-up study. In a 1999 issue of the *American Journal of Psychiatry*, the authors reported their findings on the same group of Gulf War veterans and found that anniversary reactions were a chronic problem for 66 percent of those who had a reaction at the six-year mark. Ninety-two percent of veterans who experienced an anniversary reaction had seen someone else seriously injured or killed. Symptoms of the anniversary reactions included sleep problems, irritability, experiencing intrusive memories, emotional numbness, and attempts to avoid thinking about the war.

The authors of a 2006 study in *Nursing Research* examined anniversary reactions for women who had experienced labor, including preterm birth, emergency C-sections, and excruciating pain during delivery. In these instances, the mothers developed post-traumatic stress disorder. For many of these women, their child's birthday was a time of stress instead of a time of joy. The reactions women had as the anniversary arrived were typical: irritation, sleeplessness, depression, and anxiety. Some women also experienced guilt because they wanted their child's birthday to be a time to celebrate.

Future research on anniversary reactions should go on to explore why they occur for some people and not others. It is possible that these reactions are a result of incomplete grieving. However, it is also possible that other psychological factors are at work. Only more studies will let us know.

See also: Emotional Stress; Grieving and Mourning; Holiday Stress

FURTHER READING

Kübler-Ross, Elisabeth, and David Kessler. *On Grief and Grieving: Finding the Meaning of Grief Through the Five Stages of Loss.* New York: Scribner, 2007.

Noel, Brook. *I Wasn't Ready to Say Goodbye: Surviving, Coping, and Healing After the Sudden Death of a Loved One.* Naperville, Ind.: Sourcebooks, 2008.

Schiraldi, Glenn. *The Post-Traumatic Stress Disorder Sourcebook: A Guide to Healing, Recovery, and Growth.* New York: McGraw-Hill, 2009.

■ BIOLOGY OF STRESS RESPONSES

The body's physiological reactions to stress. The nervous system and endocrine system coordinate the body's stress response. Organs such as the hypothalamus, **pituitary gland**, and **adrenal gland** are key components in the stress response. Chemicals such as **norepinephrine**, epinephrine, and **cortisol** help the body engage in the **fight-or-flight response**. **Chronic stress** can cause cortisol levels to remain high in the bloodstream, in turn causing numerous health conditions.

AN OVERVIEW

The body's response to stress is complex. Parts of the brain, the nervous system, various glands, and hundreds of chemicals are involved, yet it only takes a split second for the stress response to occur.

The **amygdala** is the part of the brain responsible for determining threats and activating the body's stress responses. The amygdala processes information gathered from the body, such as sites, sounds, smells, movements, and so forth. If a threat is perceived, the amygdala sends the information to the **hypothalamus** and other parts of the brain, at which point the stress response has begun.

THE NERVOUS AND ENDOCRINE SYSTEM

There are two systems in the body that are central to the stress response: the nervous system and the endocrine system. The nervous system consists of two major systems: the central nervous system and the peripheral nervous system. The central nervous system triggers the stress response, and the peripheral nervous system puts the response into action, specifically in the **autonomic nervous system** (ANS), one of its components. *Autonomic* means "self governing," and the ANS is responsible for the involuntary functions of the body, such as breathing and the heart's beating.

There are two systems within the ANS that help control the fight-or-flight response. The first is the **sympathetic nervous system**. This system is responsible for starting the fight-or-flight response. It is designed to expend energy and causes changes to the cardiovascular, respiratory, renal, gastrointestinal, and endocrine systems.

The other system within the ANS is the **parasympathetic nervous system**. The role of the parasympathetic nervous system is to return the body to a state of normalcy. It helps calm the body down and set the body's functions back to normal. This includes slowing down the heart, lowering blood pressure, increasing blood flow to the skin, returning the function of the GI (gastrointestinal) tract, and constricting the pupils.

The endocrine system is the other major system involved in the stress response. This system consists of glands that are located throughout the body. Examples of these glands include the pineal, adrenal, pituitary, thyroid, and pancreas. The glands secrete **hormones** into the blood. The endocrine system interacts with the nervous system. The glands most relevant to the body's stress response are the hypothalamus, pituitary, and adrenal.

Hypothalamic-Pituitary-Adrenal Axis

The hypothalamus, pituitary, and adrenal glands make up the HPA axis. The hypothalamus is the part of the brain that connects the nervous and endocrine systems. The hypothalamus regulates the body's basic needs, such as thirst, hunger, and sleep. The sympathetic nervous system is controlled by the hypothalamus. It also controls the pituitary gland. Nine hormones are produced by the hypothalamus. One hormone—**corticotropin-releasing factor** (CRF)—is particularly important because of its effect on the pituitary gland.

Corticotropin-releasing factor causes the pituitary gland to release another stress-related hormone called adrenocorticotropic hormone, which is abbreviated ACTH. The pituitary gland also releases both **prolactin** and **vasopressin**. Prolactin suppresses the reproductive system, while vasopressin helps the body retain water. **Endorphins** and **enkephalins** are released by the pituitary gland and the brain. Endorphins make people feel good and help limit the amount of pain a person experiences. Enkephalins work to suppress pain.

Q & A

Question: What does it mean when someone talks about the "chemical cascade" that happens during stress?

Answer: The chemical cascade refers to the chemical reactions in the body when stress occurs. Hormones are produced by the hypothalamus, which triggers hormones in the pituitary gland, which then triggers hormones from the adrenal glands. The corticotropin-releasing factor triggers a "cascade" of hundreds of chemicals that are released in the body due to stress.

Once corticotropin (ACTH) enters the bloodstream it causes the adrenal gland to release glucocorticoids. Although there are several types of glucocorticoids, the most abundant and important one is cortisol.

STRESS HORMONES AND NEUROTRANSMITTERS

Cortisol is the hormone many consider to be the most important in the fight-or-flight response. Cortisol increases blood pressure and blood sugar. It helps to suppress the **immune system,** provides a quick burst of energy, lowers pain sensitivity, and improves memory function. Cortisol works more slowly than norepinephrine or epinephrine. It is designed to help sustain the body's stress response if necessary.

A 2008 study in the *European Journal of Applied Physiology* presented evidence that cortisol levels change during physical and psychological stress. The authors measured cortisol levels in two groups of people. The first group engaged in exercise—cycling on a stationary bike. The second group also engaged in cycling and at the same time had to perform simple mental tasks. The physical stress (exercise) elevated cortisol levels in everyone. However, those who had to perform simple mental tasks had even higher levels of cortisol in their system. The authors explained that if this simple task caused cortisol levels to rise higher, more complex or serious tasks (such as dealing with emergencies) would produce even higher levels of cortisol.

Norepinephrine, also known as noradrenaline, is released by the adrenal gland and sympathetic nerves. This **neurotransmitter** raises blood pressure, increases the heart rate, and slows down the functioning of the GI tract, bladder, and rectum. It also dilates the pupils, draws blood from parts of the body, and directs the blood to the heart, brain, and skeletal muscles. Norepinephrine also helps convert liver **glucogen** into glucose, which is used for energy.

Epinephrine, otherwise known as **adrenaline,** is also released by the adrenal gland and sympathetic nerves. Epinephrine causes increased respiration and an increased heart rate. It also helps slow down the GI tract.

EFFECTS OF CHRONIC STRESS

The biological reactions to stress are meant to be short term. These reactions help people to tackle stressful events and then allow the body to return to its normal state. If the body is constantly in the fight-or-flight mode, short- and long-term damage can occur.

Q & A

Question: What do *homeostasis* and *allostatic load* mean?

Answer: Homeostasis is considered to be an ideal state where the body is functioning at its best. When stress hits, chemical changes produce an ideal state for the body to respond to the stress. Once the stressful event is over, the parasympathetic system shuts down the stress response, allowing the body to function properly given the circumstances (no stress). *Allostatic load* refers to the consequences the body suffers when it is forced to adapt to negative situations. When the body's stress response system is overworked, the body will suffer. The greater the chronic stress, the higher the allostatic load will be.

When levels of cortisol are constantly high, there can be negative consequences on the body. For example, a person will develop increased abdominal fat, which can lead to cardiovascular problems. Thyroid and blood sugar problems can also develop. Because the stress response lowers the body's immune system, chronic stress can keep the immune system suppressed. This can lead to illness and more difficulty fighting off infections. Further, muscles can start to deteriorate when cortisol remains in the system for too long.

OTHER CONSEQUENCES OF CHRONIC STRESS

There are additional consequences of chronic stress. The HPA axis may eventually stop working properly, causing people to become over- or under-responsive to possible threats. A 2009 study published in *Biological Psychiatry* produced evidence of this problem. The authors measured cortisol levels in teenage girls when exposed to a stressor. Most of the girls were victims of abuse and neglect. There was a control group of girls who had not been abused or neglected. The authors found the abused girls had a lower physiological response to stress when compared to the girls who had not been abused. The chronic exposure to abuse and neglect caused the body to develop a habituation effect toward stress. A person who develops the habituation effect experiences a decreased response with repeated stimulation. The body becomes desensitized to the stress.

It is important for a person to find ways to reduce the amount of stress. The body is not designed to successfully handle an extended stress response period. One way to mitigate the stress response is to have a healthy outlook about one's life. In a 2008 study in the *Journal of Personality and Social Psychology,* the authors examined how psychosocial resources, useful emotional states such as optimism and a sense of control, affect cortisol levels in response to stress. For example, the people with strong psychosocial resources are optimists, have positive self-esteem, tend to be outgoing, and feel they have control over outcomes. The authors of this study found that people with higher levels of psychosocial resources had lower levels of cortisol in their bodies when responding to stressful events.

See also: Blood Pressure and Stress; Exercise and Stress; Medication; Meditation; Stress and the Heart

FURTHER READING

Goldberg, Stephen. *Clinical Physiology Made Ridiculously Simple.* Miami, Fla.: Medmaster, 2007.

Sapolsky, Robert M. *Why Zebras Don't Get Ulcers, Third Edition.* New York City: Henry Holt, 2004.

Timmins, William G. *The Chronic Stress Crisis: How Stress is Destroying Your Health and What You Can Do to Stop It.* Bloomington, Ind.: AuthorHouse, 2008.

■ BLOOD PRESSURE AND STRESS

The pressure exerted by the flow of blood through the heart and blood vessels and how a person responds to conflict, frustration, and anxiety under that pressure. Blood pressure is one of the body's vital signs. It is a key indicator of the state of the circulatory system and overall health. For that reason, health practitioners keep a close watch on blood pressure. A doctor or nurse will measure blood pressure at office visits and routine physical exams. At hospitals, electronic monitors display a constant readout of blood pressure during surgery or while a patient is confined to an emergency room bed.

MEASURING BLOOD PRESSURE

There are different ways to measure blood pressure. The traditional way is by using a **sphygmomanometer,** along with a stethoscope. The doctor or nurse places a cuff around the upper arm and uses a stethoscope to listen to the blood pumping through the brachial artery, inside the elbow. The cuff is inflated by pumping it full of air.

This temporarily cuts off the blood flow to the arm. When the cuff is slightly deflated, the doctor hears the blood flow resume. A column of mercury in the manometer climbs along a millimeter scale, measuring blood pressure. The highest reading is systolic (maximum pressure), while the lowest is diastolic (minimum pressure). A normal blood pressure reading of an adult is 120 millimeters systolic over 80 millimeters diastolic, or 120/80.

Systolic readings over 140, or diastolic readings over 90, indicate high blood pressure, also known as **hypertension.** This can be a sign of chronic physical or psychological stress. If blood pressure remains elevated, it can lead to permanent damage to the heart and arteries, and ultimately to a fatal stroke or heart attack.

THE EFFECT OF STRESS ON BLOOD PRESSURE

One of the most important physical effects of stress is a short-term rise in blood pressure. When the body is faced with a sudden, life-threatening situation, the adrenal glands that adjoin the kidneys release certain "stress hormones," including **cortisol, adrenaline,** and **norepenephrine,** into the bloodstream. These hormones act immediately to improve strength, sharpen brain function, and raise the body's threshold, or perception, of pain. They also impair the digestive and reproductive systems, which in an emergency situation become (temporarily) unnecessary. The body prepares for "fight or flight," a throwback to prehistoric times, an instinctive reaction to escape or engage an enemy or prey.

Although encounters with wild beasts or marauding enemies are rare in the modern world, people still face stress, and bodies that were once adapted to life in the natural environment still respond with the "fight-or-flight" mechanism. Angry encounters, romantic troubles, family disputes, the loss of friends or loved ones, a final exam, or financial worries can all bring about episodes of intense stress. When they are released, cortisol and other hormones accelerate the heart rate, constrict the blood vessels, and raise blood pressure in order to bring increased blood flow to the muscles. The effects are temporary. When the danger or **stressor** passes, and the body begins to relax, stress hormones subside along with their physical effects.

CHRONIC STRESS AND HIGH BLOOD PRESSURE

A single stressful episode is not enough to permanently raise the blood pressure and bring about a serious case of hypertension. However, if there are enough stressors present to cause the frequent release of stress hormones, there could be damage done by the elevated level of these hormones in the blood. The hormones may damage the arterial walls, weakening them and causing poor blood flow throughout the circulatory system. Frequent rises in blood pressure can also put a strain on the heart and kidneys, through which the blood circulates. A permanently high level of cortisol affects the **immune system,** causes blood sugar imbalances, impairs brain function (including memory), lowers muscle mass and bone density, and adds abdominal fat, which can pose a serious health problem on its own.

People with stressful jobs are exposed to more frequent release of stress hormones. The result is a case of hypertension that can persist even when the source of stress is eliminated. The health effects include heart disease, poor digestion, frequent headaches, poor memory and brain function, and impairment of the immune system.

Individuals vary when it comes to their reaction to stress as well. The levels of stress hormones and their effect on blood pressure are part of the body's physical makeup that varies from one person to the next. These differences correlate with other attributes. People with higher cortisol levels, for example, tend to eat more and take in more carbohydrates than their low-cortisol peers.

Adults are not the only ones facing stressful episodes and high blood pressure. A year-end exam, a physical fight, arguments with teachers or friends, and disciplinary action at school can all raise blood pressure, temporarily, in young people. Also, the expectations of parents, relatives, and friends place emotional stress on young adults.

Even a visit to the doctor and a blood pressure reading can cause a brief spike in that reading. Some patients report lower BP when taking readings at home than at the doctor's office. The "white-coat syndrome" is an episode of high anxiety and stress in reaction to a medical exam.

THE RELAXATION RESPONSE

The effects of stress hormones, including rising blood pressure, lessen as the stressor disappears or fades away. Unfortunately, not all stressors conveniently vanish. Some persist: an ongoing family argument, a marital breakup, or a financial disaster such as a foreclosure on a home or a business bankruptcy. Other stressors recur at regular intervals; these might include school tests, athletic games, or even commuting daily in heavy traffic.

Some medical research has shown that constant stress situations can give rise to chronic high blood pressure. If the stressors cannot be avoided, a relaxation response can at least help the recovery and bring down the blood pressure. Here is one method:

1. Find a quiet place to sit down and relax.
2. Eliminate all outside stimuli: noise, activity, conversation.
3. Close your eyes.
4. Relax the muscles in your feet, then your legs, your arms, your chest, finally your neck.
5. Breathe steadily, through your nose. Each time you exhale, say the word *one* to yourself.
6. Continue for 10 minutes.
7. Open your eyes.
8. Sit quietly for a few minutes.

Fact Or Fiction?

Coffee raises your blood pressure.

The Facts: One of coffee's known side effects is a temporary rise in heart rate and blood pressure. However, experts disagree on whether heavy coffee drinking makes these effects chronic. The *British Medical Journal* published findings in 1991 stating that, for people with mild hypertension, restricting caffeine did not reduce their blood pressure. Similarly, in 1997, another study from the National Institutes of Health found no direct relationship between caffeine intake and elevated blood pressure. A study conducted at Duke University in 1999, however, measured blood pressure and levels of stress hormones adrenaline and noradrenaline among 72 coffee drinkers. On the days drinkers had coffee, their levels of stress hormones were higher than normal, and they remained higher well after the last cup of the day.

CONTROLLING HIGH BLOOD PRESSURE

Medical doctors recognize a blood pressure reading of 120 to 139 systolic, or 80 to 89 diastolic, as mildly high blood pressure, or prehypertension. Doctors do not typically prescribe medication for prehypertension unless the patient also has diabetes or heart disease, in which case even mildly high blood pressure can be dangerous. Instead, they advise lifestyle changes, such as lessening stress by avoiding stressors, quitting smoking, exercising every day, and following a better diet.

Stage 1 high blood pressure

Stage 1 high blood pressure occurs when the systolic reading is between 140 and 159, or the diastolic is 90 to 99. Diuretic (water) pills will help rid the body of extra water and sodium, which should help blood pressure to go down. If the condition continues, there are additional medications available. Some work by lowering or blocking production of angiotensin, a hormone that causes blood vessels to narrow. Others are beta blockers, which lessen nervous-system stimuli to the heart and circulatory system. Calcium-channel blockers reduce the effects of calcium on the smooth muscles in the heart and blood vessels, which also lowers blood pressure.

Stage 2 high blood pressure

Stage 2 high blood pressure is the dangerous kind, which can cause serious health damage to the heart, kidneys, and arteries. Patients with chronic high blood pressure have an increased risk of suffering a heart attack, stroke, kidney failure, and other life-threatening complications. Doctors will usually prescribe diuretics in combination with one or two other forms of medication. This prescription cocktail will work faster than simple lifestyle changes, or water pills alone, but such medications often cause side effects. Usually, in cases of hypertension, doctors will also prescribe a monitoring system, which allows a patient to measure his or her blood pressure several times a day.

Other methods of control

Alternative methods allow people with hypertension to control their BP without using prescription drugs. Some common methods of combating high blood pressure are simple lifestyle changes, which also make healthy common sense: losing excess weight; regular exercise; and eating a diet of whole grains, fruits, vegetables, and low-fat dairy. High levels of sodium can make blood pressure worse. A look at food labels reveals the high concentration of sodium in most packaged foods. A common recommendation is to keep sodium intake below 1,500 milligrams a day. Eliminating or lessening the intake of salt also helps, as one teaspoon of salt already contains more than 2,000 milligrams of sodium. Smoking and alcohol also increase blood pressure.

Lowering physical and emotional stress is also a good way to reduce high blood pressure. In a world of many types of family relationships, demanding school and work schedules, and constant activity, lowering stress is not always easy to accomplish. However, each person is capable of finding his or her own prescription to lowering stress, which ultimately is good for one's health. If nothing works, however, ask your doctor for help.

See also: Biology of Stress; Medication; Treatment

FURTHER READING

Larkin, Kevin T. *Stress and Hypertension: Examining the Relation between Psychological Stress and High Blood Pressure.* New Haven, Conn.: Yale University Press, 2005.

Rogers, Sherry A. *The High-Blood Pressure Hoax.* Syracuse, N.Y.: Prestige Publishing, 2008.

■ EMOTIONAL STRESS

Psychological responses to conflict, confrontation, and pressure—common components of everyday life. To some degree, emotional stress is present in any relationship. Uncertainty over the future, making deadlines at school, and concerns over money all give rise to reactions that can result in health problems if these reactions become chronic.

Emotional stress affects a majority of the population. According to the American Psychological Association's 2007 survey, "Stress in America," 48 percent of Americans believe their stress level has increased over the past five years, and one-third say they are suffering from extreme stress. The most important factors causing stress, named by three-quarters of those who experience it, are money and work.

SOURCES OF EMOTIONAL STRESS

Work is a very common cause of emotional stress. A difficult boss, a lack of control over work assignments, a sense of not being appreciated or being underpaid, and conflicts with coworkers all can lead to negative emotional reactions. Most people work in the same place and with the same people on an everyday basis, a situation that leads to a buildup of stress that becomes increasingly difficult to resolve. For adults, work stress also arises from the need to make money and support oneself and a family, a need that is constantly under threat through layoffs or a firing. A lack of satisfaction with work, or a sense that one is not suited to it, can also bring about a stress reaction.

Family problems are also a common source of stress. Siblings fight with each other; parents discipline children; couples argue over household chores, money, their relationship. The estrangement of close relatives over long distances also brings stress in the form of guilt, loneliness, or frustration. The presence of chronic stress can bring about separation or divorce and the breakup of the family.

Health problems, especially recurring illnesses or chronic diseases, also cause emotional stress. By interfering with a normal routine, and with the body's functioning, illness brings a stress response that continues until it is resolved. Illness also can make a person more susceptible to stress symptoms.

Certain people might be predisposed to respond to situations with a stress response. In a study at the University of California in Los Angeles, researchers discovered that a genetic mutation in the portion of the brain that responds to physical pain causes some people to have a stronger stress response in the case of social rejection. For those people, for example, being left out of a group or activity can literally hurt.

THE STRESS MECHANISM

Emotional stress induces a physical response in the human body. The need to take action to avoid some kind of threat or emergency causes the **hypothalamus** and pituitary gland to signal the release of **stress hormones** through the adrenal glands. The hormones temporarily increase the body's muscular strength, respiration, heart rate, and blood flow. This **"fight-or-flight"** mechanism continues to function, even though its original, evolutionary purpose—to deal with a sudden, life-threatening danger—is mostly absent from modern societies.

In the distant past, emergencies were soon resolved by escape or death. In the modern world, the human body still reacts to stress, although in the different form of unresolved issues of family, work, money, or other personal problems. Negative events can occur in quick succession—failure on a test, followed by a parent's job layoff, followed by a marital separation, followed by the need to move one's residence. All these factors might be accompanied by ongoing financial problems as well. Taken alone, each event brings stress that can eventually be resolved as one adapts and adjusts. However, together, if these types of events occur in a short period of time, an individual can lose the normal ability to cope.

The release of stress hormones still occurs, at a lesser and more continuous rate. The more **stressors** present, the more frequent is the stress response. The presence of elevated levels of **cortisol, adrenaline,** and other compounds meant to prepare the body for flight or fight brings about the common psychological and physical symptoms of chronic stress.

SIGNS AND SYMPTOMS

While physical stress affects the body directly, emotional stress has its strongest effects on mental function. Chronic stress creates tension and **anxiety,** hindering the ability to control one's thoughts or

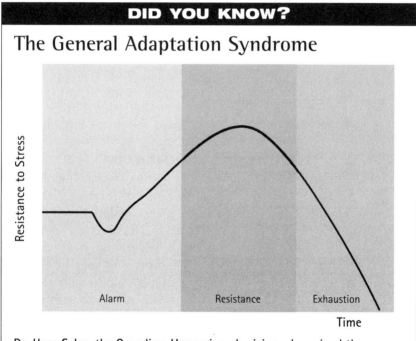

DID YOU KNOW?

The General Adaptation Syndrome

Resistance to Stress

Alarm   Resistance   Exhaustion

Time

Dr. Hans Selye, the Canadian–Hungarian physician who coined the term *stress* as it is used in modern medicine, developed the General Adaptation Syndrome (GAS) to describe how all animals, including humans, react to a stressful situation. The GAS begins with a period of alarm, followed by a peak resistance period, when the body adapts in order to cope to a continued stress. The final stage is exhaustion, in which resistance gradually fades, and the body is overcome by a range of physical and psychological symptoms.

concentrate normally. A serious case can bring a sense of panic, and long-term stress can lead to depression, in which a person finds it nearly impossible to function.

The signs of oncoming emotional stress include irritability, anger, and impatience. For a person exhibiting these emotions, even everyday problems pose serious difficulties. Eventually, people under chronic stress lose energy and begin to feel apathetic. They tend to lose track of appointments and have a hard time following normal routines. They withdraw from the outside world and avoid interacting with friends, spouses, and other family members.

The symptoms of chronic emotional stress take a toll on the body. It may become difficult for a person under stress to eat normally, and he or she may turn to junk food, or lose his or her appetite altogether. A stressed person may turn to alcohol to alleviate anxiety. Although a temporary stimulant, alcohol eventually contributes to depression and makes it even more difficult to sleep or function.

Emotional stress can bring on high blood pressure, pain and tension in the back or neck, headaches, and problems with digestion. The body seems to lose its control over heart rate and breathing and may experience a swing in temperature, from chills to sweats.

The most serious cases of emotional stress induce chronic physical problems and irrational fears. Self-destructive or dangerous, risky behavior may follow, such as thoughts of suicide or violence, as a person subconsciously seeks some kind of release from the pressure of worry and anxiety.

Q & A

Question: What's the difference between a stress reaction and anxiety?

Answer: A stress response is a reaction to a specific event. It can come from situations, thoughts, or people that are the causes of a person's uncertainty, frustration, anger, or nervousness. In a chronic state, stress can cause physical and psychological illness. Anxiety, however, is an abnormal fear that arises from the anticipation of stress, not a reaction to a specific or actual event. Anxiety can be part of a psychiatric condition such as depression, panic disorder, obsessive-compulsive disorder, or phobia.

COPING WITH EMOTIONAL STRESS

Time pressure, personal confrontations, and uncertainty over school or work or money are everyday realities for the vast majority of people. Negative events happen frequently, and stressful transitions—on the job, during a move, or within the family—are common occurrences. Even positive changes can bring some negative feelings and a sense of anxiety. Because emotional stress is always present, to some extent, in normal life, coping means tolerating and adjusting to it.

Adjusting to stress means keeping the physical body in good health and developing a positive attitude and self-image. It also requires a sense of control. If several stressful events or changes happen in a short period of time, people lose their natural ability to adapt. They expend more energy than they normally would to deal with these changes and may suffer the effects of elevated stress hormone levels.

The nature of the stress affects the usefulness of the coping strategy. Stressors that cannot possibly be changed—the ongoing relationship with a family member or supervisor, for example—demand that a person draw on support and advice from others. Problem-solving techniques are better used in stressful situations that one can change.

Lifestyle Defenses

There are several approaches available to cope with chronic emotional stress. In addition to appropriate medication, doctors usually recommend a program of regular exercise. Running, jogging, bicycling, swimming, or another aerobic workout improves health and diverts the mind, at least temporarily, from outside worries and anxiety.

In the sense that emotional stress most often arises as a result of relationships with others, these relationships can also be the key to lowering stress. Someone under stress can improve the situation by asking for help or advice from a doctor, a trusted friend, or a professional counselor. A support group is another valuable coping mechanism, as people facing the same kind of problem can share experiences and offer empathy.

Coping Distance

Another useful coping mechanism is to put the stressor at a distance, when possible. School vacations provide such distance. This also means taking a break from work, a short vacation, or finding a period for solitude in which one can reflect quietly on the problem.

The coping distance can prepare a person for a more direct action that can change the stressful situation. A period of reflection allows the mind to make decisions, without the pressures of everyday life or the immediate expectations or demands of others.

This method also helps to put the stressful situation in perspective. When stressors are up close and seem to require immediate reactions, there is a sense of urgency and great importance. When a stressor is compared to the past events of a lifetime or to long-term future prospects, however, the stressor often shrinks to a more manageable size. By gaining perspective, a stressed person can also lower expectations on him- or herself and on others.

Relaxation Therapies

Relaxation therapies also can help people deal with threats and problems. These therapies include: regular meditation, in which the body is at rest and the mind is cleared of all thought to focus on a syllable or sound; yoga, a physical exercise that takes the body through a series of balanced poses and helps to calm a person's "inner voice"; and progressive muscle relaxation, in which groups of muscles are tensed then relaxed. This last therapy also helps a person recognize the onset of physical stress and deal with it when it becomes frequent or chronic.

Counseling

Seeking professional counseling is of course a useful coping mechanism. Psychotherapy allows a patient to communicate the events of his or her life and talk about conflicts and problems. It is especially useful when dealing with relationship problems, family matters, and social anxieties.

Holistic counseling involves both the physical body and the mind. It allows an individual to use various therapies to help create a sense of well-being in both a physical and psychological sense.

Prevention

Although emotional stress cannot be avoided completely, there are ways to better prepare for it. These include keeping close friendships with others, in which support is available if needed. Maintaining a healthy routine, getting enough sleep and maintaining an adequate diet, regular exercise, avoiding abuse of alcohol, drugs, or stimulants such as caffeine, all help people prepare for dealing with life's stressors. Many doctors also recommend periods of rest and relaxation during the day to stop the constant flow of demands on the body and the frequent need to make decisions.

See also: Stress Management Techniques; Treatment; Types of Stress

FURTHER READING

Bradberry, Travis, and Jean Greaves. *Emotional Intelligence 2.0.* San Diego, Calif.: TalentSmart, 2009.

Charlesworth, Edward A., and Ronald G. Nathan. *Stress Management: A Comprehensive Guide to Wellness.* New York: Random House, 2004.

Groves, Dawn. *Stress Reduction for Busy People: Finding Peace in an Anxious World.* Novato, Calif.: New World Library, 2004.

▣ EXERCISE AND STRESS

Doctors and stress researchers generally agree that an exercise program can counteract the physical and mental effects of stress. Exercise also can help people to better cope with stress as well as to prepare their bodies for episodes of **acute** stress that occur from time to time.

PHYSICAL AND MENTAL BENEFITS OF EXERCISE

Episodes of stress bring about the release of certain hormones into the bloodstream, which prepare the body for physical action in the face of immediate danger. This "fight-or-flight" reaction is useful in helping the body deal with a life-threatening situation. However, constant, low-level, chronic stress does more harm than good. Stress hormones raise the heart rate and blood pressure, raise the production of glucose, suppress the immune system, shut down the digestive process, and divert blood away from the skin and extremities to the major muscle groups and most essential organs of the body. If stress continues, all of these effects eventually will damage the body, causing major illness, fatigue, and loss of brain function.

Exercising counteracts the effects of chronic stress. It creates a series of beneficial chemical reactions within the body. If done on a regular basis, these changes provide some immunity to the harm done by chronic stress and the release of **stress hormones** such as cortisol and **adrenaline** into the bloodstream. Exercise also improves the function of muscles, organs, and the **immune system,** helping the body to better cope with an illness or injury.

Fighting or Fleeing

When exercising, the body is actually carrying out the actions—"fight or flight"—that the stress hormones are designed to help. As far as the body knows, a person exercising is "fighting" or "fleeing," only without the immediate physical danger. He or she may be running, jogging, bicycling, speed walking, or taking part in team sports, martial arts, or some other physical contest with an opponent. Someone who exercises is using up stress hormones, returning the body to its normal chemical balance and helping to eliminate stress hormones from the system.

Letting Out Anger

Exercise is also a safety valve for the release of built-up anger or hostility. This is especially important because in modern societies a physical expression of anger is not usually acceptable. When anger or **anxiety** is kept within, chronic stress builds up, affecting the immune system and making the body more vulnerable to illness. Exercising that allows some form of physical contact, such as boxing or martial arts, is especially effective at releasing anger and in learning to control hostile responses.

Brain Changes

When the body is put through a physical workout, the supply of blood and oxygen to the brain increases. This improves mental function by helping to clear away certain **toxic** chemical compounds that can build up in the brain and make it difficult to think and process problems.

Research has also shown that physical exercise concentrates the release of **norepinephrine** into the brain. This **neurotransmitter** helps to control the release of stress hormones into the bloodstream during a stress response. With the enhanced release of norepinephrine, exercise helps the different systems of the body coordinate their response to episodes of stress. Chemically speaking, people who exercise deal with stress more effectively and efficiently than those who do not.

Happy Endorphins

In 1996, the surgeon general of the United States issued this report: "Physical activity appears to relieve symptoms of depression and anxiety and improve mood." Researchers agree that vigorous exercise stimulates the release of neurotransmitters known as **endorphins,** natural substances that are produced by the pituitary gland and the **hypothalamus.** Endorphins are useful to the body by helping to block the sensation of pain, which is transmitted by the body's nerve endings. Endorphins also create a feeling of exhilaration and well-being and can help to counteract some of the physical effects of stress hormones.

Release of Muscular Tension

When someone fails to exercise, the muscles and tissues build up toxic substances as well as what is known as "resting tension." The inactivity robs muscles of their healthy tone and potential for work. Physical exercise allows the muscles to release the tension, condition themselves, build up fiber and mass, and better prepare for hard work, if necessary. Sedentary people often complain of aches and pains in muscles as well as joints. It might be difficult to understand why muscles ache if they do not have any work to do, but the explanation is simple enough: Muscles at rest gradually lose their conditioning and will respond with pain if subjected to even slight stress, such as poor posture or sleeping in an uncomfortable position.

Fact Or Fiction?

Exercising builds muscles.

The Facts: The physical work of exercise stimulates an increase in muscle mass, which takes place when the body is at rest. If you exercise every day, without taking a break between sessions, you are not allowing this period of recovery and are slowing muscle development.

Diverting Stress

Exercise also helps people affected by stress by focusing the mind on the physical activity at hand. Riding a bicycle, for example, takes a certain amount of concentration and mental focus: to keep the body balanced, to prompt the arms and legs to their proper action, to follow a given route, and to avoid obstacles. These necessary functions temporarily relieve the mind of worry about a stressful situation. In turn, this can help the **subconscious** mind work on the problem and arrive at a solution, without conscious effort or prompting.

The repetitive motion of many forms of physical exercise also helps the brain attain a calm and focused state similar to that achieved through meditation. The work undertaken by the body during exercise—steady and deep breathing, movement of the limbs, regular bending and stretching—synchronize brain and body functions.

Exercise also helps you sleep. When the body is physically tired through repetitive activity, a person more readily falls asleep and can achieve deeper and uninterrupted sleep throughout the night. The ability to sleep well is one of the main weapons in the fight against stress.

Social Benefits

Exercise also increases general well-being and defeats stress by helping an individual achieve goals. Concentrating on the number of laps swum in a pool, for example, and surpassing a previous "personal best" can bring an enhanced sense of self-worth and control that can be carried over to combat episodes of stress because loss of control in any situation is one of the most common causes of stress.

Another benefit of exercise is the enhanced **self-esteem** that comes with improved physical conditioning and appearance: Both are products of a regular exercise program. Self-esteem and social acceptance are directly related to the ability to cope with stress, whether at home, on the job, or at school.

When exercising, people may either work out alone or in a group. Either environment can bring benefits. A period of solitude while working out can allow one to temporarily escape a stressful situation. Playing a team sport such as softball or basketball, or a one-on-one competitive exercise such as racquetball or tennis, can help one to bond with others, make beneficial physical contact, and reduce the sense of isolation that contributes to chronic stress.

Exercise allows people to become more sensitive to changes in their muscles and other parts of the body. Researchers refer to this ability as "somatic awareness." An individual in good shape is keenly aware of his or her heart rate, rate of breathing, muscular tension, and other physical attributes. This helps them to sense the physical warning signals of chronic stress and prompt them to take positive steps to overcome those symptoms. Some people in poor shape may be less aware of the unhealthy physical changes that are the result of an increase in stress.

Benefits of Competition and Cooperation

Physical exercise can mean keen competition with others, a calculation of risk, and facing physical danger. When a person is regularly engaged in such activities, he or she is better able to handle the mild stressors of everyday life. Long lines in the cafeteria, heavy traffic at rush hour, or losing a set of keys become mild annoyances, not stress episodes. To a certain extent, the body can condition itself psychologically to suppress the stress response, control the release of stress hormones, and save the wear and tear and fatigue that these hormones cause over time. Competition and cooperation with others in a sports environment enhances the ability to resolve stressful situations in other environments.

AN EFFECTIVE EXERCISE ROUTINE

To be effective in combating stress, an exercise routine should be fun—not work. Individuals have their own preferences when it comes to exercise and should tailor their exercise to these preferences. For some, jogging is an enjoyable exercise, and for this reason it is effective in improving their physical and mental well-being. For others, jogging is boring; imposing a jogging routine on themselves would just cause a sense of obligation and drudgery—another form of chronic, low-level mental stress.

Competitive sports can be an effective way to exercise, but overly competitive situations can bring anxiety in preparation and anticipation of the match, and a sense of guilt and letdown in the case of defeat. A sense of competition with oneself also can be a source of anxiety; constantly striving to better a personal best time in swimming or biking is not likely to help a chronic worrier or someone afflicted with stress symptoms. Exercise should promote a sense of self-esteem, and people should compete with others who are at or near their skill level. This will help defuse the pressure to perform that can come from team sports.

Most doctors recommend **aerobic exercise** as the most effective at combating stress, or combining aerobic and anaerobic workouts. An aerobic exercise such as walking or swimming works the body at a steady pace, increasing the heart rate and respiration and gradually conditioning the muscles and joints. Anaerobic exercise works the muscles hard to build strength. As in weightlifting or pull-ups, it is usually carried out in a series of sets or repetitions.

The frequency of exercise determines its effectiveness. Frequency is more important than intensity; the body cannot make up for lack of

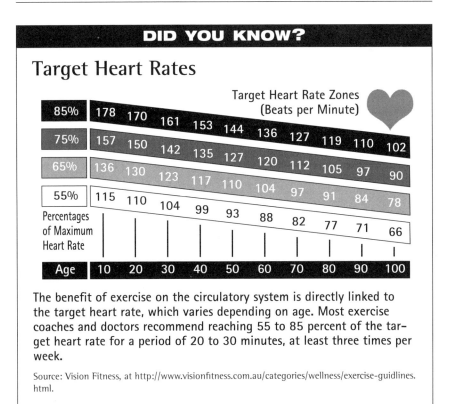

DID YOU KNOW?

Target Heart Rates

Target Heart Rate Zones (Beats per Minute)

Percentages of Maximum Heart Rate										
85%	178	170	161	153	144	136	127	119	110	102
75%	157	150	142	135	127	120	112	105	97	90
65%	136	130	123	117	110	104	97	91	84	78
55%	115	110	104	99	93	88	82	77	71	66
Age	10	20	30	40	50	60	70	80	90	100

The benefit of exercise on the circulatory system is directly linked to the target heart rate, which varies depending on age. Most exercise coaches and doctors recommend reaching 55 to 85 percent of the target heart rate for a period of 20 to 30 minutes, at least three times per week.

Source: Vision Fitness, at http://www.visionfitness.com.au/categories/wellness/exercise-guidlines.html.

exercise by a longer or more intense session of physical work. Some amount of exercise, as brief as 20 minutes, is recommended every day, at least to prepare for the longer sessions that occur less frequently.

Of course, exercise is best when done in moderation, and not by compulsion. Some people may exercise so often, and so diligently, that they suffer physical symptoms or emotional upset if they miss a session. Like some other basically healthy or positive behaviors, exercise can become an addiction. When this happens, stress may arise when the routine is interrupted, defeating one of the most important reasons for exercising in the first place.

See also: Stress Management Techniques; Treatment

FURTHER READING
Locke, Marius, and Earl G. Noble. *Exercise and Stress Response: The Role of Stress Proteins.* Boca Raton, Fla.: CRC Press, 2002.

Wilmore, Jack H., David L. Costill, and W. Larry Kenney. *Physiology of Sport and Exercise.* Fourth Edition. Champaign, Ill.: Human Kinetics, 2008.

■ GENDER AND STRESS

The different physical and emotional ways in which males and females respond to events that upset one's balance. Men and women experience different physical effects from stress episodes, and they also have different ways of coping with stress.

REACTION TO STRESS

The difference in how men and women react to stress has been widely studied since the middle of the 20th century. Most studies have found a significant difference in stress responses between the genders. In one study at the University of Pennsylvania, researchers placed men and women in a stressful situation and found that different areas of the brain are activated in response to a stressful event.

The research suggests that the brains of men and women may have taken a different evolutionary path. Over the millennia of confrontations and external **stressors,** males and females developed a different response, one that eventually affected the structure and functioning of their central nervous systems. In males, the "fight-or-flight" reaction, the instinct to either confront or flee a danger, is stronger. Females, on the other hand, react to stress by "tending and befriending," by nurturing their young and forming social alliances to meet a common danger. By forming such alliances, the chance of survival of a larger group of people under dangerous conditions is improved.

Sensitization

Another interesting result of laboratory research is the study of witnessed stress and sensitization. In the search for a stressor that might affect men and women somewhat equally, researchers at the Rosalind Franklin University of Medicine and Science selected the Holocaust, a massive genocide in which more than 11 million people were murdered, including the extermination of 6 million Jews. The Holocaust took place in territory under the control of Nazi Germany during World War II (1941–45). The results of the Holocaust were partially documented in film when Nazi concentration camps were liberated by the Allies in 1945. They found bleak prison camps, starving and tortured prisoners, mass graves, and indescribable human suffering. The Rosalind Franklin researchers exposed their male and female subjects to these horrifying films on two different occasions, then measured changes in heart rate and negative affect, the feelings or impressions as reported by each subject.

The results show that women were gradually sensitized to the scenes they witnessed and displayed significantly more intense effects than did men on the second showing. Women also reported intrusive thoughts and "avoidance," or the attempt to avoid thoughts of stress suffered by others, in the interval between the screenings.

The results suggest that women may be more prone to **anxiety**, depression, and negative thoughts following exposure to a stressful event. Men seem to have greater ability to accustom themselves to stress; women do not accustom themselves as readily and overall have a greater susceptibility and higher rate of anxiety and depression, which in turn may be as a result of their different physical and psychological reactions to stress.

STRESS TYPES

Males and females also show a difference in the type of stress that most seriously affects them. In a study published in *Biological Psychiatry* in 2002, Dr. Laura Stroud and other researchers measured the release of the hormone **cortisol** in men and women when faced with different kinds of stress. The results suggested that men react more strongly to "achievement" stressors, in which they are under stress to accomplish a task or perform, either physically or mentally, in competition with others. Women react more strongly to social rejection and to uncertainty in their place among the members of a group.

Boss Stress—Male and Female

Researchers also have looked at the gender of individuals *causing* stress, and the different effect males and females have when serving as the source. In 2005, researchers at the University of Toronto used a phone survey of workers in the United States to study men and women working either for a lone male boss, a lone female boss, or for one male and one female boss. The results showed that women suffer more anxiety, depression, and other symptoms when working for a single female boss. There was no difference among men, however: Male and female single bosses caused about the same stress-reaction symptoms.

The results were also different for the mixed pair. In working for a female and a male, women experienced more stress than when working for a male only. Men who worked in the same situation experienced less stress than while working for a single male.

The results suggest, among other things, that female workers, at least, may have different expectations for their bosses. These expectations arise from the different roles taken by the genders in society. Women may be expected to be more cooperative, supportive, and nurturing than men, whose more aggressive leadership tactics accustom workers to their bossy behavior. A lack of traditionally feminine qualities in a female boss, therefore, brings about a higher level of stress in female workers. For some reason, men do not make the same distinction as employees: Both female and male bosses stress them out at about the same level.

The Stress of Work Expectations

Many studies have brought about the conclusion that men and women bring different hopes and expectations to the workplace. The differences are not exclusive. Men focus on pay, promotions, status, and achievement; they are more likely to seek leadership positions and authority over coworkers. Women value such things as well but also see the workplace as a place of social relationships and place higher importance on communication with others, the respect of their peers, and collaboration. Men react more negatively to situations where they have less control; women object to being isolated.

Not understanding the different expectations generally true of the different genders can lead to higher stress in the workplace. Women, in general, experience higher levels of stress on the job than do men. Part of the reason may be that many occupations were, at one time, held exclusively by men and developed a male-oriented culture. Such occupations may not be as congenial to female employees, who experience higher rates of stress as a result.

The pressures of the job market have their effect on men as well as women. Difficulty finding a job, the danger of losing one's job, lack of promotion, and stagnant wages cause stress in men with families, who are expected to provide support as the principal breadwinners. In troubled economic times, employed workers respond by working longer hours, taking less vacation time, and suffering higher levels of stress. The fatigue brought on by long hours of work also tends to make people more sensitive to stressful situations encountered outside of the job and may bring on physical and mental health problems as a result.

OTHER DIFFERENCES

Out in the wider world, away from school or work, the differences in reactions to stress between men and women continue. In addition to experiencing a higher level of stress, women in general seem to have a larger number of concerns to worry about: not just work but also family and relationship issues, financial problems, the state of their homes, their friendships, and their relatives. Men seem to worry less often and about fewer things, and when they do the emphasis is on work and money.

Internal Pressure

Men and women also place different kinds of stresses on themselves in reaction to the demands of the outside world. Girls and women tend to sacrifice themselves to the needs of others, while boys and men strive to surpass personal goals. Women tend to react to this stress by making connections with others, while men enjoy escape, often to physical activity, for example, or to "down time" in isolation from the sources of their stress and anxiety.

Social Isolation

Researchers have also suggested that growing social isolation may be playing a role. With the advent of easy travel from one city to the next, and more frequent job changes, women are more likely to find themselves in a new place, lacking friends and family. Without their accustomed support networks, they suffer more from the emotional stress that arises from family, health, and job problems.

Differences in the body's reaction to stress also play a role in the different responses of men and women. The release of stress hormones proceeds differently in men and women. In a stressful situation, both genders will produce **cortisol** and **adrenaline,** the **stress hormones** that cause raised blood pressure, faster pulse, and other reactions to prepare the body for "fight or flight." In women, however, a calming hormone known as **oxytocin** is released in greater quantities and has the effect of countering the physical and emotional reaction to stress hormones. Even as women may be subjected to more stressors, more frequently, than men, their bodies are adapted to overcome or cope with that stress more quickly. By relaxing the body, oxytocin also contributes to the "tend and befriend" reaction seen more commonly among women.

Both sexes are suffering the health effects of higher levels of chronic stress. Instead of occasional emergency situations that required an immediate response, modern men and women are dealing with low-level stressors that are more frequent and long-lasting. The result is a higher concentration of stress hormones in the body, which in some cases leads to anxiety, depression, sleeplessness, and high blood pressure. In the contemporary world, people face less physical danger but more serious health problems from the phenomenon of chronic stress.

TEENS SPEAK

I Talk It Out

My brother and I are the same age and go to the same school, but they don't let us go to the same classes. I think his courses are a lot easier than mine. I take science and math, and I did a lot better on the SATs this year than he did. My parents want me to go to college and get a degree and get ready to be a doctor or a lawyer. That means a lot of hard work right now to get good grades. For my brother, they don't put on that kind of pressure. "We expect a lot from your sister," they tell him, and leave it at that.

I don't get why everything seems easier for him. When I have a paper due or a test coming up, I can't sleep well and I worry a lot about it. If he gets worried, he just seems to keep it all inside. But I don't think he worries too much. Sometimes he asks for help studying or for the answer to a question. For some reason I want to help him out if I can. If we talk about a problem, sometimes he comes up with the answer on his own.

If I need help, forget it. He doesn't want to talk about it. He just tells me I'm smart enough to figure it out on my own. Or he might just make a guess. I guess that makes him feel like he tried, anyway.

That's when I just call one of my friends in the same class and work it out with her. We can talk about the problem and about other things that are going on. Usually the phone call goes for about a half-hour. I probably wouldn't call a guy I knew, even if I thought he knew the answer. Guys never want to talk it out.

Stress and the Young

Doctors, psychologists, and researchers all recognize the different gender responses to stress among teenagers and young adults. Researchers also verify that students in high school experience higher stress levels, in general, than adults. In addition, female students tend to be more stressed than males. The sources of stress are more numerous, self-esteem is generally lower, and the social pressure of peers is more keenly felt. As young people grow older, the sources of their stress also change, from school issues to job and money matters. Girls also have an additional source of stress in the worry over personal safety. They feel less safe than boys in the halls of their school or in the streets of their neighborhoods.

Studies also show that as teenagers become adults and begin taking on adult tasks of finding work and starting families, their stress tends to ease off somewhat. The constant search for a place among friends and family, and in society at large, continues to affect teenagers until some of the important questions about their futures are answered.

See also: Anniversary Reactions; Emotional Stress; Stress and the Family; Types of Stress

FURTHER READING

Gray, John. *Why Mars and Venus Collide: Improving Relationships by Understanding How Men and Women Cope Differently with Stress.* New York: HarperCollins, 2008.

Kimmerling, Rachel, ed. *Gender and PTSD.* New York: The Guilford Press, 2002.

Nelson, Debra L. *Gender, Work Stress, and Health.* Washington, D.C.: American Psychological Association, 2002.

▧ GRIEVING AND MOURNING

The intense sorrow people experience from the loss of a loved one and the public expression of that grief. The death of a spouse or close family member is one of life's most stressful events. Grieving brings a period of **anxiety** and physical and emotional stress that can be hard to overcome. Physical changes overtake the body that are related to the chemical reactions triggered by the "fight-or-flight" response.

In evolutionary terms, this kind of loss represents a threat to survival: Early humans lived in small groups, with each member of the group dependent on the others to secure food, shelter, and protection against enemies. When a member of a close family group dies, a sense emerges in the group of a heightened threat from the surrounding world. This triggers a physical response—more **acute** in cases of sudden or accidental death. Because there is no escape, no "fight or flight," from the loss of a family member, an unresolved sense of **chronic** stress begins. Stress related to grieving can last for weeks or months and can cause serious illness or even death.

The grieving process can arise as a result of events other than death. These might include a broken romance, the loss of a friend, the loss of a job, even the loss of a favored possession with deep sentimental value. Many people are familiar with the sense of grief over a lost pet; others have experienced chronic stress and depression over the defeat of a favorite sports team or a personal failure in some competition. Researchers have found several common threads running through these different causes of grief, depending on the nature of the loss and the psychological makeup of the individual who suffers that loss.

ANTICIPATORY GRIEF AND SUDDEN LOSS

In an age of high-tech medical care, many people can survive for long periods with terminal illnesses or be sustained in a coma or a disabled state for years before dying. This delay can cause a case of "anticipatory grief" in family members and friends, anticipating the loss of a loved one. Feelings of guilt over the past relationship, as well as the sense that more should be done, can contribute to chronic emotional stress. The hard decisions that must be made on continuing life support or administering medication cause additional anxiety. Death may be inevitable, but its time may be uncertain, which causes heightened anxiety and even feelings of detachment from the dying relative.

The state of Oregon has made extensive studies of families dealing with chronically or terminally ill members. The Oregon Health Services have found that those forced to make life-or-death medical decisions experience more long-term stress. Researchers in Oregon have also studied the effects of assisted suicide (legal under that state's Death with Dignity Act) and found that family members who experienced this process did not suffer more periods of prolonged grieving. The reason, the researchers speculated, was that these families have time to prepare for the death and are therefore relieved of the uncertainty surrounding the end of a prolonged or terminal illness.

Sudden loss of a loved one through an illness, accident, suicide, or some other cause brings shock, disbelief, and a feeling of confusion. The sudden death leaves the relationship permanently broken, with no way to resolve issues between someone who has passed away and those left behind. The grieving person may suffer an episode of acute stress at hearing the news or witnessing the death. This can cause mental confusion, sleeplessness, anxiety, and depression, all symptoms that may return each year in what is known as **anniversary stress.**

STAGES OF GRIEF

During the 1960s, Elisabeth Kübler-Ross, a Swiss-born doctor and researcher into the phenomenon of grieving, identified five major stages of grief: denial, anger, bargaining, depression, and acceptance. Many grief counselors and psychiatrists still follow this structure, although it has come under questioning by more contemporary grief researchers, and other "stage theories" also exist. People have different social and cultural traditions, and so the grieving process varies among individuals, although the stages (sometimes appearing in a different order) are readily identifiable.

Denial

The sense of disbelief on hearing the news of a death begins the first stage of grief: denial. For some time, the mind cannot accept the loss and a numbing disconnection from the outside world is the result. Someone in denial over a loss may believe that a mistake has been made, that the deceased has been wrongly identified, or that he or she is living through a bad dream from which the person will soon wake up.

Anger

When denial is no longer an option, a sense of anger sets in directed against oneself or against someone or something else. A person who is experiencing the pain of a loss may lash out against family members, caregivers, doctors, or anyone perceived to share responsibility for the death. The anger may eventually turn against the deceased, who is blamed for the sense of loss and abandonment. Finally, it can turn inward; it is common for grieving people to examine their own past

DID YOU KNOW?

The Modified Grief Cycle

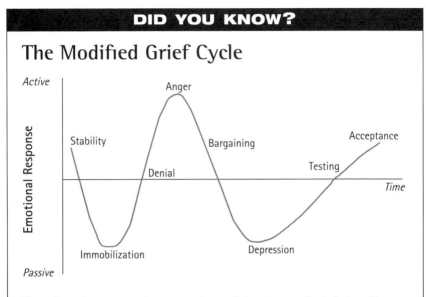

There have been many interpretations of the stages of grief since it was first proposed by Elisabeth Kübler-Ross in *On Death and Dying.* In this chart, passive and active emotional responses alternate as a person moves through the stages of grief, which have been expanded to include "stability," "immobilization," and "testing."

Source: http://changingminds.org/disciplines/change_management/kubler_ross/kubler_ross.htm

actions and try to think of what else they could have done to prevent the death.

Bargaining

From anger, persons grieving often turn to bargaining. They attempt to strike a deal in order to come to terms with their loss, to live a better life, and to put off their own mortality. They will turn to outsiders who they believe can help them. Bargaining can take the form of religious devotion, of resolutions for personal change, or a drastic change in one's relation to others.

Depression

The loss of hope brings a sense of deep sorrow and the realization that recovery from grieving will be a long and difficult process. This can be a prolonged period of anxiety and depression; in this stage, people find it difficult to resume work or a normal life, or even keep up daily habits such as eating, sleeping, or grooming. They may drop friend-ships and contact with family members and become lonely, sensing that no one else can understand their feelings. A sense of "survivor's guilt" may develop, causing one to question why he or she should be alive when a loved one is dead.

Acceptance

In the final stage of grief, the mourner reaches a point of acceptance. He or she comes to understand the permanence of death and the need to recover some form of ordinary life. The emotional struggle with guilt and sorrow begins to pass; the sense of being under constant physical and mental stress also begins to ease. The griever resumes home and work routines, seeks out friendships again, and may turn to the society of others who have experienced the same thing. By the time this stage is reached, several months or years may have passed.

GRIEF AND EMOTIONAL STRESS

The grieving process can bring on a case of chronic stress. A person suffering a personal loss can experience feelings of helplessness, sad-ness, anger, and loneliness. Behavior may become strange or antiso-cial. He or she may experience periods alternating between depression and a sense of euphoria. In extreme forms, this kind of stress can lead people to harm themselves or others. The mental impairments can include a loss of affect, the absence of any reaction to others or to surroundings. Thinking can become disorganized and difficult. People who are grieving may attempt to shut out the sense of loss by becom-ing obsessed or focused on an idea or small detail of their lives.

Visual and auditory hallucinations are also common during periods of grief and mourning. The voice of the deceased may be heard or his or her presence in the room detected. People may be uncertain how to react in the presence of others or how to behave in public or with strangers. Some people's grieving becomes completely passive, and they lose interest in what's happening around them. They also may shut out all memory of the deceased and suffer a case of severe for-getfulness. They lose interest in work, hobbies, friendships, or family. Grieving can break up friendships and end marriages.

There are several variables that affect the reaction to loss. Unan-ticipated, sudden death often brings a more acute stress response than does anticipated loss. If someone has experienced a loss in the past, he or she may be even more strongly affected by another episode. If the loss has come about through an accident or by a violent act, emotional stress can include a sense of insecurity and vulnerability.

The death of a child is particularly hard on parents and siblings. A young person's sudden death makes less sense than the death of someone ill or elderly, and it can take much longer to comprehend and accept. In one study at the Columbia University School of Nursing, researchers gathered information on 74 parents who had lost children and found that 60 percent of these individuals were still in the process of grieving nearly 20 years after the death. However, the commonly held view that the death of a child inevitably leads to the breakup of the parents was contradicted by a 1999 study, *When a Child Dies*, by the Compassionate Friends group and has not since been refuted. The group found that 72 percent of marriages had survived the death of a child and that only 12 percent ended in divorce—a lower rate than that for marriages in general.

Fact Or Fiction?

If you lose a friend, you just have to be strong.

The Facts: Losing a friend who has moved away, or with whom you've had a fight, can be a painful experience and cause a grieving process. Allowing yourself to recognize that you are grieving and letting out your fears and your feelings will help you get through it more quickly.

PHYSICAL STRESSES OF GRIEVING

Grieving has many different effects on the body. The release of **cortisol** and other **stress hormones** into the bloodstream increases. The brain and nervous system are stimulated, causing a rush of images and thoughts. Sleeplessness often results, and vivid dreams and nightmares are common. A grieving person loses the ability to concentrate or perform any kind of mental work. Heart rate becomes irregular, breathing sometimes shallow, and blood pressure rises. The digestive system is affected, making it harder to digest and eliminate food. A grieving person can become chronically angry and irritable or unfocused and unable to pay attention to anything. He or she may lose the ability to carry out simple, ordinary actions or follow habits they once did without even thinking about them. Loss of coordination can make a grieving person accident-prone; fatigue can become a constant companion. The stress of grieving can make one more vulnerable to illnesses, including heart disease, ulcers and other digestive problems, skin conditions, and more serious diseases such as kidney failure and cancer.

RESOLVING GRIEF

Grief is a process of healing the mind and body after a loss. Through the grieving process, the body slowly returns to a state of equilibrium after the stress caused by a strong emotional shock. This can take different lengths of time for different people, and it also depends on relationships with others, past experience with grieving, and the positive steps taken to deal with grief.

There are several methods of overcoming grief and resolving the stress it brings. Psychologists and counselors usually advise someone who has experienced a personal loss to take some time off and lessen his or her workload. They recommend following a regular and healthy diet, doing some form of daily exercise, and reserving some periods of time for simple rest.

As much as possible, people who are grieving should suspend the busy daily schedule and make their lives less burdensome. This means canceling appointments that are not urgent, putting off travel, and not making any long-range plans. A loss of energy is a typical reaction to grief, and placing the body under further physical and mental stress will extend the time needed for recovery.

For many people, grieving and mourning never resolve. Reminders of the loved one, anniversaries, and random memories can trigger a return of grief symptoms. Some people are better adapted to overcome these effects than others. The researcher Mary Frances O'Connor at the University of California in Los Angeles studied 23 women who had lost a mother or daughter to breast cancer and who had experienced either complicated (long-lasting) or noncomplicated (resolved) cases of grief. O'Connor showed pictures of the lost family member to their subjects while scanning different portions of the brain. She found that the group with complicated grief had greater activity in the nucleus accumbens, an area of the brain associated with social relations and attachments, and with sensations of yearning and longing. As activity in the nucleus accumbens has the effect of "rewarding" the brain, the "complicated" grievers may be psychologically "addicted" to the memory of a loved one.

The body and the mind react to grief and loss in complex ways that are still the subject of intense research. As medicine slowly extends the average life span, overcomes once-fatal diseases, and forces people into difficult life-or-death decisions, the issue of grieving remains the subject of ongoing questioning and debate.

See also: Anniversary Reactions; Emotional Stress; Stress and the Family; Types of Stress

FURTHER READING
Fitzgerald, Helen. *The Grieving Teen: A Guide for Teenagers and Their Friends*. Fireside, 2000.
Kübler-Ross, Elisabeth, and David Kessler. *On Grief and Grieving: Finding the Meaning of Life Through the Five Stages of Loss*. New York: Scribner, 2007.
Worden, J. William. *Grief Counseling and Grief Therapy: A Handbook for the Mental Health Practitioner*. New York: Springer, 2008.

■ HOLIDAY STRESS

Physical and psychological responses to events that upset one's psychological balance during holiday periods. Holiday stress is experienced during the Thanksgiving and Christmas seasons. The end of every year brings **anxiety** to many. The expectations of friends and family and the demands of the holiday season—social and financial—can be overwhelming. Instead of a time of celebration, the holidays become for some a time to be dreaded, an ordeal to be survived.

The need by many to carry out the numerous social rituals of the season may cause a **chronic stress** level that endures for several weeks and peaks in the last week of the year. On the Holmes and Rahe stress scale, which correlates the degree of stress with the occurrence of various life events, Christmas rates a 12, between "Vacation" at 13 and "Minor Violation of Law" at 11. A study by researchers at the Mayo Clinic in Olmsted County, Minnesota, found the rate of suicide lower than average on Thanksgiving and Christmas—but higher than average, at 41 per 1 million people, on New Year's Day, the end of the holiday season.

Many factors contribute to the experience of holiday stress. For example, nearly everyone who is not a child is expected to offer gifts, resulting in the pressure to shop, spend money, and often incur debts in order to meet that expectation. Anxiety about the reception of gifts also causes stress, as givers often worry about the reaction of the recipients. If the receiver appears disappointed or indifferent, another cause of self-doubt, frustration, guilt, and anxiety appears.

In addition to gift giving, the blatant commercialization of a religious holiday causes some spiritual stress. The onslaught of advertisements in every medium also may cause feelings of fatigue and despair. For many, a spiritual vision of Christmas clashes with the commercialization that is prevalent in society. Christmas has become a time of materialism and selfishness rather than a reaffirmation of faith. Non-Christians also may become stressed or made anxious by Christmas celebrations in which they take part reluctantly or not at all.

FAMILY RELATIONSHIPS

For many families, the holidays are also a time to reunite. Family members may stay together under the same roof for a few days. Unaccustomed to the close contact, they may feel awkward in one another's presence. This can be especially true if new spouses or friends are introduced. As is natural, families often will review their experience of the past—both good and bad. This can bring former problems and personality conflicts again to the surface.

Family relationships can be fraught with tension and uncertainty. Members of the family, in reuniting, may be seeking approval or consolation, while children may be going through a period of intensified **sibling rivalry.** The loss or absence of a spouse, parent, or child can be more keenly felt during the holidays, when better times together are remembered. This can bring on a feeling of stress and depression and even result in physical responses such as loss of appetite, fatigue, and minor illnesses that find opportunity against a weakened **immune system.** Researchers at the Headache Institute at Roosevelt Hospital in New York have also found that the 30 million people in the United States prone to migraine headaches have them about 50 percent more frequently during the holidays. The causes include lack of sleep, poor diet and overeating, and increased emotional stress.

Caregivers in hospitals and hospices for the seriously ill experience family stress firsthand. Theresa M. Stephany in a 1993 commentary entitled "Holiday Stress," written for the *American Journal of Hospice and Palliative Medicine,* describes the common wish or expectation that an aged or ill relative survive for an additional Thanksgiving or Christmas. Also, a death in the family around the holidays will be a source of **anniversary stress** in the future, in which grieving worsens near the date of a loss.

Nostalgia for past holidays may place emotional stress on those who see themselves unable to re-create the magic of childhood memories, either for themselves or their children. Feeling stressed is the reaction to high expectations, the desire for the best presents, the fear of disappointment, and the ultimate letdown when the holidays are over.

TEENS SPEAK

Christmas Is Coming, and I'm Stressing Already

Every year, my family has to have a big holiday party. Sometimes we have relatives come to stay with us. Friends come over and hang out on Christmas Eve. Everyone opens presents and says how it's just what they wanted. The house is noisy, and I always have to be careful what to say and do. I can't just go out, even though I'm on a school vacation and I should be having some fun.

The worst part is having to pretend to be cheerful and happy to see everyone. That's okay for one day, but after a few days, it's impossible. People just annoy me. And Christmas seems to get longer every year. Now we're putting up lights after Halloween, and shopping for presents before Thanksgiving.

The whole thing seems like a lot of pressure to buy stuff you can't afford, look like you're happy, and talk to your relatives. At least when Christmas Day comes around, the house gets a little quieter and that means it's almost over. By that time, I just want to shut the door and keep the world outside my room.

FINANCIAL STRESS

The holidays cause financial strain for many people. A reunion with family or friends in a distant place requires expensive, stress-filled travel, when the airports and highways are busy. Buying gifts to satisfy the wish lists of children and relatives empties out the bank account or requires people to incur credit card debt that may take a long period of time to repay. Worry about money and savings is a key component of stress and is especially severe around the holidays.

At the New Year, many people take stock of their finances. This means an accounting of how much they earn, how much they spend, the amount of their savings, the safety of their accounts, and what their money goals are. Another part is the accounting at the end of the year and the beginning of the new one on progress toward meeting financial goals and developing financial security. The postholiday financial stress syndrome has been blamed for a rise in bankruptcies at the beginning of the year.

Resolutions made at the New Year often involve goals for earning and saving. These can spur positive action or linger as additional mental and physical stress placed on workers who feel they should spend even longer hours in productive work. Expectations of children for Christmas gifts can cause additional family conflict and worry on the part of parents and their offspring. Spending money on gifts is tied closely to emotions that are difficult to control: the desire to please, nurture, and support children in their ambitions.

The holiday financial stress is especially severe for those who have lost their jobs or had their pay and hours reduced at work. For the unemployed, Thanksgiving and Christmas are sources of worry and frustration, reminders of better holidays in the past.

BIOLOGICAL STRESS

The near-constant activity during the holiday season places a great strain on the body and nervous system. People generally eat more, and many drink more. Holiday sweets, heavy meals, alcohol, and desserts add pounds and worry over weight gain. In a study conducted at the National Institutes of Health in 1999–2000, researchers weighed 195 people over a span of eight weeks, in the "preholiday," "holiday," and "postholiday" periods. The results showed an average weight gain of 1.05 pounds (0.48 kilograms) from September to February. The experiment also revealed that the participants tend to keep holiday weight gain throughout the year.

In addition to overeating and poor diet during the holidays, another example of a biological cause of stress is a lack of fitness. Together, poor eating and being in poor physical shape can lead to a weakening of the immune system, at a time of year when illnesses such as colds and flu are more common. Also, absenteeism from school and work is more common during and shortly after the holiday season because some people see the traditional days off as a time for recuperation from stress built up throughout the year. Finally, the transition back to everyday schedules also can cause physical stress on the body that has experienced holiday activities, altered sleep patterns, and nonstop socializing.

POSTHOLIDAY STRESS

After New Year's Day, the holiday season ends. For most people, life returns to normal; school is back in session, and the workplace returns to regular hours of operation. However, a mental letdown also occurs, as the holidays may have passed without bringing improvement in work, family, or financial situations. The celebrations, reunions, gatherings, and gift giving have come and gone, and the result is that things are back to the way they were before.

There are a variety of **stressors** present in the postholiday season. Households have to return to order and assimilate new possessions, and decorations must come down. These are common sources of avoidance and procrastination, which create feelings of guilt, another source of stress. Bills arrive that must eventually be paid. For many, a feeling of emptiness or loneliness arrives, placing emotional stress on those who spent a few weeks enjoying themselves.

To avoid the postholiday stress syndrome, doctors and researchers have recommended clearing out the home of unwanted or unused items. Making small steps toward returning the home to normal can help relieve postholiday anxiety. Also, stress management techniques such as meditation and regular physical exercise can help.

See also: Anniversary Reactions; Emotional Stress; Stress and the Family; Types of Stress

■ MEDICATION

Prescription drugs to reduce stress. Depending on the degree of stress, a person may need to use medications known as antidepressants to help treat depression and **anxiety disorders.** These medications work on chemicals in the brain called **neurotransmitters. Serotonin,** dopamine, and **norepinephrine** are the key neurotransmitters.

All medications have side effects, ranging from minor to serious. Although one serious concern about some antidepressants is the possibility that they increase the likelihood a person may think about or attempt suicide, research does not support this concern. In fact, when someone is suffering from a clinical depression or anxiety disorder, the risks of not taking medication are much greater than the risks of side effects associated with proper treatment.

ROLE OF MEDICATIONS IN STRESS MANAGEMENT

Antianxiety and antidepressant medications are commonly prescribed for the treatment of symptoms associated with stress. The National Institute of Mental Health (NIMH) estimates that approximately 40 million people in the United States suffer from an anxiety disorder in a given year. The institute also estimates that more than 12 million women and 6 million men suffer from depression in a given year.

The authors of a 2009 article in the *Archives of General Psychiatry* state that antidepressants are the most commonly prescribed class of medications in the United States. There is obviously a significant need for antidepressants because many people cannot relieve their symptoms with other types of therapy alone.

NEUROTRANSMITTERS AND STRESS

Antidepressants work by targeting chemicals that influence anxiety and depression. These chemicals are referred to as neurotransmitters. Neurotransmitters can be thought of as chemical messengers in the brain. They allow cells to communicate with one another and play an important role in learning, mood, memory, pain perception, sleep, and a multitude of other physical and mental functions. According to the Australian Academy of Science, hundreds of neurotransmitters have been discovered.

Neurotransmitters play a key role in the body's ability to handle stress. Three neurotransmitters are critical to depression and anxiety disorders: serotonin, dopamine, and norepinephrine. Although other chemicals also play a role, these three neurotransmitters are the ones targeted by medications.

SELECTIVE SEROTONIN REUPTAKE INHIBITORS

One of the most widely used classes of antidepressants are the **selective serotonin reuptake inhibitors** (SSRIs). The first SSRI appeared on the market in 1987 with the brand name Prozac (generic: **fluoxetine**). Since then, numerous others have been developed. They include **sertraline** (Zoloft), **fluvoxamine** (Luvox), **citalopram** (Celexa), **escitalopram** (Lexapro), and **paroxetine** (Paxil).

All of these drugs are designed to make more serotonin available to the brain. It is believed that insufficient amounts of serotonin are

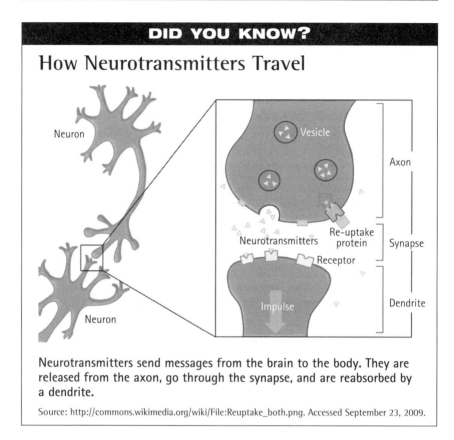

How Neurotransmitters Travel

Neurotransmitters send messages from the brain to the body. They are released from the axon, go through the synapse, and are reabsorbed by a dendrite.

Source: http://commons.wikimedia.org/wiki/File:Reuptake_both.png. Accessed September 23, 2009.

responsible for depression and anxiety disorders. These medications help prevent serotonin from being reabsorbed into various nerve cells (called receptors). The increased amount of serotonin helps improve mood.

There are seven different types of serotonin receptors in the body. The reason there are a variety of SSRIs is that each works slightly differently on the receptors. Therefore, if one medication does not work, others can be tried.

Several side effects are associated with SSRIs. These include restlessness, weight gain, insomnia, nervousness, nausea, sexual dysfunction, agitation, headache, dry mouth, and diarrhea. Unfortunately, sometimes restlessness, nervousness, and agitation can result from taking a medication designed to help alleviate anxiety and depression.

A more serious side effect is called **serotonin syndrome**. This rarely occurs, but when it does it can be fatal. Serotonin syndrome occurs when an SSRI interacts with other medications or supplements that are designed to raise serotonin levels. Signs of serotonin syndrome include seizures, extreme agitation, confusion, hallucinations, fever, elevated heart rate, and fluctuations in blood pressure.

SEROTONIN AND NOREPINEPHRINE REUPTAKE INHIBITORS

Serotonin and norepinephrine reuptake inhibitors are another class of medications that help with anxiety and depression. These medications work to increase both serotonin and norepinephrine levels in the brain. Medical experts believe that targeting two neurotransmitters can help with these conditions if an SSRI is not working. However, it is ultimately a doctor's decision to try SNRIs later in the treatment of depression or at the outset.

There are two SNRIs available for use: **duloxetine** (Cymbalta) and **venlafaxine** (Effexor). The side effects of these medications are the same as those for SSRIs. There are some additional side effects, including problems with vision, tremors, gas, and having abnormal dreams. Serotonin syndrome is also a possibility with SNRIs.

NOREPINEPHRINE AND DOPAMINE REUPTAKE INHIBITORS

Norepinephrine and dopamine reuptake inhibitors (NDRIs) are designed to keep more norepinephrine and dopamine in the brain by blocking their reabsorption. Although there are more than 10 different types of NDRIs, only one is used for depression. That is **bupropion,** also known as Wellbutrin.

Bupropion has some different side effects than do SSRIs and SNRIs. Side effects can include skin rash, lack of appetite and weight loss, ringing in the ears, muscle and stomach pain, anxiety, sore throat, and increased urination. Other side effects include sweating, nausea and vomiting, agitation, constipation, dizziness, and seizures.

TRICYCLIC ANTIDEPRESSANTS

Tricyclic antidepressants (TCAs) were developed before SSRIs. They prevent both serotonin and norepinephrine from being reabsorbed into various receptors. Doctors usually prescribe the newer generation of medications before trying a tricyclic antidepressant.

There are eight different TCA medications: **amoxapine, amitripty-line, desipramine, doxepin, imipramine, nortriptyline, protriptyline,** and **trimipramine**. Each has a slightly different chemical structure; if one does not work, a doctor can try using another.

Side effects of TCAs are similar to those found with SSRIs and SNRIs, namely weight gain, constipation, dry mouth, increased appetite, and nausea. These medications also can cause blurred vision and urinary retention, low blood pressure, and sensitivity to sunlight.

TETRACYCLIC ANTIDEPRESSANTS

There are two tetracyclic antidepressants (TeCAs) that doctors may prescribe to help reduce the stress associated with depression: **maprotiline** and **mirtazapine**. These medications work differently than the other antidepressants. Instead of preventing the reabsorption of norepinephrine and serotonin, these medications do not allow the neurotransmitters to bind with nerve cells.

Tetracyclic antidepressants have many of the side effects of other medications, including weight gain and increased appetite, dry mouth and thirst, dizziness, drowsiness, constipation, and increased cholesterol.

MONOAMINE OXIDASE INHIBITORS

Monoamine oxidase inhibitors (MAOIs) have been used since the 1950s to help treat depression. As with TCAs and TeCAs, they are not typically used as a first line of treatment but rather when other medications fail. These medications help all three neurotransmitters maintain high levels in the brain.

There are more than 20 different medications that are classified as an MAOI. Four have been specifically approved by the Federal Drug Administration (FDA) for the treatment of depression: **phenelzine, selegiline, isocaboxazid**, and **tranylcypromine**.

Monoamine oxidase inhibitors are associated with an extensive list of side effects: drowsiness, dizziness and light-headedness, constipation or diarrhea, fatigue and weakness, low blood pressure, restlessness and trembling, increased appetite and weight gain, trembling, muscle twitching, and shakiness. Although these appear to represent the "standard" list of side effects found with antidepressants, there is a more serious concern with MAOIs: These medications can interact with certain types of food and drinks, resulting in dangerously high blood pressure and possible stroke. People on an MAOI have to eliminate or seriously limit the amount of food they consume that contains a chemical called tyramine. Tyramine can be found in many alcoholic beverages such as beer and wine. It also can be found in some types of meat, chocolate, cheeses, and pickled foods.

BENZODIAZEPINES

Benzodiazepines are medications designed to help with anxiety and sleep problems. They are the most common medications used to treat the stress that results from anxiety. These drugs act as minor tranquilizers by slowing down the central nervous system. This produces feelings of calmness and relaxation in people taking these medications.

According to the U.S. Drug Enforcement Administration, there are 15 different types of benzodiazepines available in the United States, with an additional 20 available in other countries. Some of the most commonly prescribed include **lorazepam** (Ativan), **alorazolam** (Xanax), **diazepam** (Valium), **clonazepam** (Klonopin), and **chlordiazepoxide** (Librium).

Unlike the other medications discussed in this section, benzodiazepines do not focus on serotonin, dopamine, or norepinephrine neurotransmitters. They influence the neurotransmitter gamma-amino butyric acid (GABA). GABA neurotransmitters influence the body by slowing or stopping the nerve impulses. Benzodiazepines enhance GABA's ability to do its job. As a result, people become more relaxed and may become sedated.

The side effects that people can experience include confusion, lack of motor coordination, impaired memory and thinking, slurred speech, altered vision, nausea, constipation, vomiting, diarrhea, and respiratory depression. If benzodiazepines are taken in high doses, people may also experience mood swings, euphoria, and erratic behavior.

Benzodiazepines are not meant for long-term use. It is estimated that after four to six months of regular use, a benzodiazepine loses its effectiveness. The medication can lose it effectiveness sooner if the body develops a tolerance for it. If this happens, the person may need a higher dose to achieve relaxation or sleep. Long-term use can cause people to be cranky, have headaches, be depressed, have troublesome dreams, and have no energy or interest in normal activities. The most significant problem with long-term use is the possibility of **addiction.**

Benzodiazepines are highly addictive. Addiction can occur within a few weeks. If addiction becomes an issue and the medication is stopped abruptly, a person can suffer from withdrawal symptoms, including shaking, sweating, convulsions, insomnia, more anxiety, confusion, paranoia, muscle aches or spasms, and flulike symptoms.

Even if a person tapers off the use of the medication, withdrawal symptoms may occur.

Q & A

Question: Do illegal drugs affect neurotransmitters?

Answer: Yes, part of the reason illegal drugs make people feel good is due to their immediate effects on neurotransmitters. For example, the illegal drug ecstasy works on serotonin. It causes serotonin to be released, blocks it from being reabsorbed, and depletes serotonin levels in the brain. Long-term use damages the cells that make serotonin, reducing the amount of serotonin available to the brain. If a person is on an antidepressant and takes ecstasy, there is a chance of experiencing serotonin syndrome.

MEDICATIONS AND SUICIDE

Much controversy surrounds the possible link between taking antidepressants and attempting or committing suicide. There are many misconceptions about this link. In 2004, the U.S. Food and Drug Administration (FDA) instructed U.S. drug manufacturers to add a warning to the labels of all antidepressants. The warning indicated that there is an increased risk of suicidal thinking or suicide attempts by children and adolescents who take antidepressants. In 2007, the FDA had this warning include people up to the age of 24.

The authors of a 2007 article in the *American Journal of Psychiatry* pointed out that the evidence the FDA used to determine the need for warnings suffered from major limitations. The FDA looked at data from randomized control trials of antidepressants. They found that youth taking antidepressants were twice as likely to engage in suicidal thinking or behaviors. However, there were no suicides among the youth studied. For adults, the FDA found eight people committed suicide who were in studies of antidepressants. However, three of the suicides were by people taking placebo pills or a control medication. The remaining five people who committed suicide were among the 53,030 patients taking an antidepressant.

More research

Research on the link between antidepressant use and suicide has shown that there is very little connection between the two. Authors of a 2009 study in the *Journal of Affective Disorders* found the use of citalopram was not related to suicidal thinking. In particular, it was discovered that the medication was unlikely to cause thoughts of suicide unless the person had such thoughts at the beginning of treatment. More important, over 50 percent of patients with suicidal thoughts before starting the medication had actually improved within two weeks of starting treatment. There was improvement by most patients at the end of 12 weeks. Fewer than half of 1 percent (0.47 percent) attempted suicide during the course of treatment. Of these cases, 52 percent had attempted suicide prior to treatment. The overall results indicate that it is very unlikely that using citalopram will lead to suicidal thoughts or suicide attempts.

A 2009 study published in the *European Journal of Clinical Pharmacology* also provides evidence that the use of antidepressants does not lead to suicide. The authors found that people over the age of 10 who were taking SSRIs were less likely to commit suicide than those not taking an SSRI or those who started taking the medication and then stopped.

Thoughts of suicide
It is important to remember that people who are severely depressed may think about suicide but not have the motivation or energy to carry through on the thoughts. Taking an antidepressant will help give people more energy as they start to feel better. However, depression does not disappear immediately once medications are started. Those who are severely depressed may start to develop enough energy to follow through on their thoughts and commit suicide. This does not mean the medication caused the suicide. Those who attempt or complete suicide are often the high-risk patients who displayed these thoughts or behaviors before starting treatment.

See also: Biology of Stress; Emotional Stress; Treatment

FURTHER READING
Breggin, Peter. *Medication Madness: The Role of Psychiatric Drugs in Cases of Violence, Suicide, and Crime.* New York: St. Martin's Griffin, 2009.
Karp, David A. *Is It Me or My Meds? Living with Antidepressants.* Cambridge, Mass.: Harvard University Press, 2007.
Libal, Joyce. *Antidepressants and Suicide.* Broomhall, Pa.: Mason Crest, 2007.

■ MEDITATION

A practice of mental focus and physical relaxation that in many people helps to relieve stress. Meditation is based on several Eastern religious philosophies such as Zen Buddhism that seek to attain a higher state of awareness by eliminating conscious thought. The attainment of spiritual enlightenment through a meditative state such as prayer or the repetition of a sacred creed is an aspiration among other religions as well. Although meditation is grounded in religious thought, many of its modern practitioners do not associate it with religious study, worship, or observance. There are many different methods of meditation; while some follow traditional teachings, others are developed outside of any training by an individual practitioner.

DAILY MEDITATION

One common type of meditation helps some people to relieve the stresses that accumulate during the typical day. For this daily meditation, there is no equipment needed and no formal instruction necessary. The session can take place in or outside the home, requiring only a quiet environment and a few moments without work or home chores, communication with others, or outside stimuli.

A person meditating must relax the body, steady the breathing, and focus all attention on a single word or sound. This mantra is repeated aloud or silently. By focusing on a single syllable, the most basic form of thought and communication, the train of jumbled thoughts that constantly strives for attention is temporarily halted. The daily information overload that burdens many people is put aside, and for a time the mind is relieved of the need to take action or consider the many exterior stimuli that bombard it. Worries over the future are suspended, while regrets over past actions can be, temporarily at least, forgotten.

For many, the short daily meditation session results in a sense of renewed calm and well-being, mainly by allowing the mind to view exterior stimuli (including worries and **stressors**) from a different perspective. The benefits of meditation can carry through as well, making meditation one of the most effective stress-management techniques.

There are many health benefits of meditation in addition to the relief of stress. In an online article on the subject, researchers from the Mayo Clinic report that depression, **anxiety, binge eating,** high blood pressure, allergies, and heart conditions are just some of the physical illnesses that a regular practice of meditation in combination with traditional treatment may help to alleviate.

FORMS OF MEDITATION

Many different forms of meditation include one of the most common and popular, **guided imagery**. Helped by an instructor, the meditator contemplates a single image, or series of images, of a place that inspires a feeling of calm and well-being. This visual memory can be enhanced with remembered sounds or smells. After the meditation session ends, a person can sometimes return to guided imagery when confronted by a stressful situation in order to more clearly understand that situation and deal with it in a positive manner.

Fact Or Fiction?

Yoga is a religion.

The Facts: Yoga is a system of guided exercise and meditation, not a religion and not a religious ceremony. It originated in India, where it was closely associated with Hinduism. As the practice of yoga spread around the world, however, it lost its religious roots and developed into a method for training the body and mind outside of any religious doctrine or belief.

Mindfulness

An alternative to guided imagery is the practice of mindfulness, in which the participant focuses on the body's immediate physical sensations such as breathing and the heartbeat. In this form of meditation, one receives exterior stimuli but tries to halt the mind's processing and judgment of those stimuli, whether they consist of noises, smells, variations of color and light and dark, or the sense of touch and texture. In addition, the usual inner distractions—emotions, fatigue, boredom, restlessness—are deliberately shunted aside.

Exercise and Meditation

Meditation is also used in connection with certain physical activities. In a yoga class, for example, the students assume various positions under the guidance of an instructor. The physical effort and concentration required as the students hold and change positions leads to a meditative state of mind, allowing calmness as well as greater concentration.

Yoga sessions are usually ended with a short session of meditation or guided imagery. Another form of exercise that employs a meditation technique is tai chi, a Chinese practice in which the person assumes a series of positions, steadily changing from one to the next with absolute concentration and steady, deep breathing.

PHYSICAL EFFECTS OF MEDITATION

Typically, meditation has immediate physical effects, including slowed pulse, lower blood pressure, and slowing the release of common **stress hormones** such as **cortisol** and **adrenaline**.

Meditation, according to one theory, might have a direct effect on the action of important regions of the brain, including the amygdala and the **prefrontal cortex.** While the amygdala helps trigger the "fight-or-flight" response and the release of stress hormones into the bloodstream, the prefrontal cortex is the center of the brain involved in rational decision making. A person well-practiced in meditation, according to the theory, would be more adept at using the prefrontal cortex in controlling sudden instinctive actions, and thus be able to lower the various physical and psychological side effects of stress.

Researchers have found that people who engage in meditation tend to develop more gray matter in the brain and to have lower incidences of dementia, Alzheimer's disease, and other illnesses common among the elderly. Experienced meditators also benefit from increased gamma-wave activity in the brain, which helps the brain achieve more concentrated states of awareness.

TEENS SPEAK

I Learned to Relax

Everyone I know hates final exams. It can mean half of your grade, and sometimes means passing or failing the course. I can study for months and I still don't feel ready. The night before, I cram a little more. Then I go to bed late and can't sleep.

I figured out one way to deal with it. After I wake up, I just sit in a chair for about 10 minutes. I close the door, so nobody bothers me. I don't think about the test. I just look out the window. There's a street out there, but not too busy. Cars pass by from time to time, in one direction or another. I think about where they might be going.

I think about myself on that road. I'm driving along and going someplace else. Somewhere that I like to be. Usually it's a park I know about 10 miles from town. There's a lake there for swimming, and it's good just to walk around the trails for a while. You can cook some food on the grills and relax, do nothing. When I'm sitting there, the sounds outside my window seem the same as the sounds I'm hearing in the park. The voices I hear on the sidewalk belong to people in the park, enjoying themselves. When I get totally relaxed, it feels as if I'm about to fall asleep. That's when I wake up and get to it.

By the time I'm at school, sitting down, taking the test, I'm ready for it. If I get nervous about an answer I just clear out my head for a minute and go back to the park. When I do this, sometimes the answer will come into my head.

It seems to work pretty well.

STRESS REDUCTION AND MEDITATION

Medical research has shown that meditation induces many stress-reducing reactions in the body's nervous system. In 2008, researchers from the University of Oregon took part in a large study of meditation in China. The study compared two groups of students: an experimental group using meditation and a control group in which participants were going through simple relaxation training. Before and after five days of training, the Oregon researchers gave the students a series of mental tests, designed to induce a stress reaction. The study found the group going through meditation training to have a much milder stress response, including a lower level of cortisol, the stress hormone, than those in the relaxation training control group. The control group also had higher levels of anxiety, fatigue, and anger. This and other studies have found that meditation may limit activity in the sympathetic nervous system, which is responsible for the stress response.

In another study, at the Keck Laboratory at the University of Wisconsin, researchers examined the brain waves of two groups of meditators: eight Tibetan monks who had practiced meditation for at least 15 years and 10 student volunteers. Brain scans showed both groups producing high-frequency gamma waves while meditating, with the monks producing a far higher concentration and coordination of these waves, which are associated with stronger memory, concentration, and learning.

In other studies, meditation also has been found to reduce anxiety, lessen the incidence of chronic depression, and relieve the symptoms of post-traumatic stress disorder. Attention deficit disorder also has been treated with regular meditation sessions as has seizure disorder, also known as epilepsy, because the use of meditation can reduce the stress and anxiety that can bring on seizure episodes.

In a study published in the medical journal *Integrative Cancer Therapies,* researchers attempted to understand the effect of meditation on a group of breast cancer patients 55 years of age and older. By reducing stress (one factor in the development of breast and other cancers), meditation improved the patients' quality of life and emotional well-being. Although the use of meditation and the reduction of stress may seem irrelevant to a serious and complicated medical condition such as cancer, many studies have linked mental function and emotional states with the body's disease-fighting abilities. Through mechanisms that are still under study, it seems that a daily practice that allows the mind to focus on inner processes rather than exterior distractions also can improve the basic immune functioning of the body.

See also: Emotional Stress; Medications; Stress Management Techniques; Treatment

FURTHER READING

Bharati, Swami Veda. *Meditation: The Art and Science.* New Delhi, India: Wisdom Tree, 2008.

Rama, Swami, Rudolph Ballentine, and Alan Hymes. *Science of Breath: A Practical Guide.* Honesdale, Pa.: Himalayan Institute Press, 2009.

Wallace, B. Alan. *Contemplative Science: Where Buddhism and Neuroscience Converge.* New York: Columbia University Press, 2007.

■ PERFORMANCE ANXIETY

A feeling of heightened stress and foreboding in anticipation of a difficult task, such as speaking in public. Performance anxiety is familiar to athletes, musicians, and anyone who must perform before a group of people. It also can occur in the intimate moments between two people preparing for a sexual encounter. Along with emotional responses come physical symptoms such as rapid heart rate, shallow breathing, tension in the muscles, and higher blood pressure. All these are caused by the release of **stress hormones,** including **adrenaline,** into the bloodstream. The natural "fight-or-flight" syndrome moves into operation, prompted not by a direct encounter but by anticipation of the event, as well as fear of failure, defeat, or humiliation.

AMONG PERFORMERS

Musicians, singers, and actors all face performance anxiety as a part of their professional life. For most people, no matter how capable or naturally talented they are, the thought of performing a difficult task in front of a large audience induces an abnormal sense of self-consciousness, anxiety, physical discomfort, and emotional stress. For those who appear in public on a regular basis, performance anxiety becomes a familiar and constant fear, something to cope with by calming routines, actions repeated before each performance that over a long period of time become automatic and help to relieve the stress.

Stage Fright

All actors have experienced stage fright, and some of the most famous actors in the world never quite get over it. Laurence Olivier was an English actor considered by many the greatest Shakespearean performer of the 20th century. The Oscar-winning Olivier acted in hundreds of plays and movies and was known for his cool, calm, serious demeanor. However, a paralyzing stage fright sometimes affected him, even when performing in roles he had known and memorized for decades. During some performances, he had to ask his fellow actors never to look him in the eye, claiming that this made him forget his lines. In one performance of *Hamlet,* a bout of anxiety erased Olivier's memory of the most famous soliloquy in all of Shakespeare's works; he could not even recall the line, "To be or not to be!" While the audience waited, he simply sat down onstage until the speech came back to him.

Other Public Performances

An athlete may prepare for a game by doing a simple calisthenic routine, dressing slowly and methodically, and then visualizing the kind of play he or she needs to win a victory. The repetition of familiar actions successfully completed helps to calm the mind. It lessens the sense of worry and works the muscles into a loose and flexible state, better preparing the athlete for the running, shooting, or catching to come.

All professional performers have spent many years training them-selves for their work. They must master all the technical aspects of their profession: for a musician, an instrument; for a speaker or an actor, the voice and gestures. They must have an innate feel for timing and a sense of empathy with their audience, qualities that are difficult to teach and learn. They must also develop courage, the ability to conquer performance anxiety and the apprehension that one is either unprepared for or unworthy of public acclaim. Because the mind is much more difficult to control than the body, for many performers this turns out to be the most difficult part of their job, and one that prevents many talented, hardworking people from pursuing a per-forming career in public.

In some forms, performance anxiety becomes stage fright, a fear that appears immediately before the concert or play begins, and which prevents a good performance. There are cognitive (mental) and physi-ological factors. Cognitive factors affect the mind, which develops a fear of errors or memory loss and a sense of inadequacy. The physio-logical factors, brought on by a release of stress hormones, can include dizziness, sweaty hands, "butterflies" in the stomach (caused by con-stricting blood vessels), and a pulse racing out of control. All these factors make the muscles, particularly in the hands, difficult to con-trol, a symptom that is deadly for most kinds of musical performance.

Researchers studying performance anxiety have found that females seem to suffer from this type of stress more severely than males, and older people less so than younger people. With experience, profes-sional performers learn to anticipate the physical stress and anxiety that arises and channel it into mental focus and physical energy. This is making successful use of the stress hormones that otherwise might lead to mistakes and a poor performance.

Also, the difficulty of a task is directly related to the degree of performance anxiety experienced; the presence of an audience also makes a difference, depending on its size and on whether the audi-ence is composed of known people or strangers. Many researchers have concluded that environment is the key source of human behav-ior and psychology. Large public audiences—particularly of strang-ers—improve the performance of a well-learned task and inhibit the performance of a poorly learned one. This is because performance of difficult learned tasks is directly related to a sense of self-confidence that is reinforced by the approval of others. A performer who has mas-tered a speech or piece of music and who also has an innate sense of the mood and reactions of an audience has taken the most important steps to lessening performance anxiety.

Q & A

Question: I have to make a presentation to my class next week, and the more I think about it the more nervous I get. What should I do?

Answer: Focus on the task at hand. Research your topic so you know it better than anyone else. Take notes, ask questions of your teacher, and read. These are all things you can do without an audience. Outline your presentation, step by step, to break it down into manageable parts that are easy to remember. Rehearse your speech in front of one classmate, then have him or her ask you questions and review your performance.

It also may be that naturally anxious people feel driven to seek the acclaim and approval that are offered in public to successful performers. Researchers have noted, for example, that musicians experience stress more acutely than nonmusicians. However, the link between performance anxiety and personality is one type of the familiar chicken-or-egg problem. The need to perform may be an outgrowth of the musician's or actor's personality, but a state of constant anxiety may also be a result of the demands of performance.

PERFORMANCE ANXIETY IN PRIVATE

Performance anxiety also occurs on a more personal, intimate level among small groups of people, or between two individuals. A meeting at work may involve convincing a group of strangers to accept a proposal or purchase a service. The presenter must make a convincing case, answer questions readily, and appear enthusiastic. This kind of private performance can induce serious mental stress, especially when employment or an entire career is at stake.

Examinations

For many students, weekly tests or final exams bring an **acute** case of stress. Negative physical and psychological responses are not uncommon when taking standardized tests for college admissions or the comprehensive tests used in states such as Florida, which are used to grade the performance of individual schools. One study by the Institute of HeartMath and Claremont Graduate University followed 980 10th-grade students and found that 61 percent were affected by test anxiety occasionally and 26 percent were affected often or most of the time. Students with test anxiety scored on average 15 points lower, in both math and language-arts examinations. The anxiety that builds up as the exam date approaches can interfere with preparing for it. Trying to cram too much information into one's memory while the body suffers the ill effects of a stress reaction can lead to sleepless nights, headaches, an upset stomach, and other reactions.

Many strategies are available to deal with test anxiety. Students can spread out their preparation over several nights or weeks and give themselves enough time to master information. Frequent review of the information also helps.

Physical readiness is as important as mental preparation. This requires getting enough sleep and exercise in the days before a test. Showing up with plenty of time to get settled also helps. When the test is placed on one's desk, a student should review the entire test first, read the directions carefully, and ask the teacher any questions that arise at the outset. Also, to avoid the pressure of time, plan for each section, moving along when necessary and not getting hung up on a difficult question. Skimming the test for simple answers first is another good technique for time management.

Job Interviews

A job interview, similarly, involves a very personal performance, one that is very difficult to prepare for. Interviews with strangers in an unfamiliar human resources office are especially stressful. One's basic competence, experience, and appearance are all under close examination. With no technical skill on display, the interviewee/performer must rely on self-confidence, memory, and a strong empathy or understanding of the interviewer: what he or she wants or expects to hear.

Ambition may have led the applicant to reach for a demanding position, but one for which he or she feels unqualified. A lack of confidence worsens the usual preperformance stress. A negative feedback loop begins: the less confidence in or mastery of a task, the lower the performance ability and the greater the anxiety in anticipation of that performance. Because many job interviews end in failure, the memory of past interviews may condition a person for a poor performance and increase the anxiety when preparing for a future interview. "Adaptive anxiety," however, allows for greater mental and physical awareness and enhances performance, whether in an interview or onstage.

Sexual Relations

Performance anxiety can also occur during sexual intimacy. Anticipation of sex can induce a release of stress hormones into the bloodstream. This can lead to performance anxiety, in which a person is unable to achieve the aroused state necessary or desired for sexual relations.

This kind of stress arises from a fear of failure and of disappointing an audience of one: a sexual partner. Blocked by anxiety, a person finds himself or herself overly focused on achieving "success" in various actions and losing the ability to act spontaneously. A stressful environment is created that inhibits the expression of true feelings and desires.

Sexual performance anxiety can damage self-esteem and ultimately destroy a relationship, especially one still in the early stages. The memory of past failures can reinforce the problem; a couple may avoid sex altogether or experience a strong and stress-inducing sense of personal rejection.

Performance problems of this sort do not always arise from an anxious mental state. A temporary dysfunction in men or women can arise from physical illness, fatigue, the use of alcohol, or problems in the home or workplace.

COPING WITH PERFORMANCE ANXIETY

Avoiding stressful situations, if possible, is one method of coping with performance anxiety. Of course, this option is closed to musicians, actors, athletes, and anyone else who needs to perform before an audience. Such performers have developed many different ways to cope. One method is a session of warm-ups before the performance, done, if possible, in front of spectators. Many musicians begin their programs with easier pieces in order to get their voices or fingers limber and to get comfortable in front of the public.

Other methods of coping with performance anxiety are simple, everyday options that have little to do with the skill on display. These include the following:

- Wear comfortable clothes and shoes onstage.
- Stick to a special "calming" diet to relieve the effects of stress on the digestive system. This diet includes easy-to-eat food such as green salads, soup broth, and fruits such as bananas and apples.
- Spend time in rehearsal. In rehearsal, actors commonly perform before small groups of strangers, whose faces and reactions are easy to read. This allows performers to get a feel for the effect of their words on an audience and condition them to the emotional "environment" of the work they are performing.
- Play a false note, which all musicians naturally fear but is not seen as a "mistake" in rehearsal, rather an incorrect method of playing: a less good alternative. Banishing the concept of "mistake" can help lessen the fear of it occurring.
- Simulate the physical effects of stress while practicing music. To do this, musicians purposely raise their heart and breathing rate (by riding a stationary bicycle, for example, or rapidly climbing stairs). They then attempt to control these distracting physical symptoms while practicing.
- Practice **guided imagery,** or moving the inner focus of performers from themselves to the music and ultimately to the pleasure of the audience. Losing the sense of self, temporarily, is often effective in reducing the inner turmoil and anxiety of a performance situation.

Other methods of coping with performance anxiety include common stress management techniques such as meditation, breathing exercise, and yoga sessions. Artificial means exist as well, including the use of **beta-blockers,** which overcome the effects of stress hormones such as adrenaline. However, as with any medication, the body may gradually build resistance to the effect of beta-blockers if they are taken on a regular basis for an extended period of time. Also, with the regular use of beta-blockers, one might develop another form of anxiety: fear of failure without medication. Alcohol is another dubious method of coping with performance anxiety; while it can temporarily boost self-confidence, it also affects the motor skills and inhibits memory and brain function.

Many performers have also turned to psychological counseling in an effort to cope with performance anxiety. Some counselors work on the assumption that performance anxiety is a response that can be unlearned. One method is to introduce someone experiencing intense anxiety to the performing environment and then instruct him or her in meditation, breathing exercises, hypnotic suggestion, or guided imagery techniques that help the person to relax. Another method is to bring negative thoughts or fears to the surface by verbalizing them, then dismissing them with words or images of a good outcome: a successful performance, a satisfied audience, a standing ovation. The idea is to condition the mind to a positive experience, even before the performance begins.

See also: Meditation; Relaxation Therapies; Stress Management Techniques; Treatment; Types of Stress

FURTHER READING

Berry, Mick, and Michael Edelstein. *Stage Fright: 40 Performers Tell You How They Beat America's #1 Fear.* Tucson, Ariz.: See Sharp Press, 2009.

Goode, Michael I. *Stage Fright in Music Performance and Its Relation to the Unconscious.* Marina del Rey, Calif.: Trumpetworks Press, 2003.

Maisel, Eric. *The Performance Anxiety Workbook.* New York: Back Stage Books, 2005.

Roland, David. *The Confident Performer.* New York: Heinemann, 1997.

■ RELAXATION THERAPIES

Different mental and physical techniques for lessening stress symptoms. Relaxation therapy is a field of study that is relied on by many doctors and psychologists to treat stress among their patients. Some relaxation therapies rely on traditional approaches such as meditation, hypnosis, and physical exercise. Others rely on the power of the mind to control the functions of the body.

MENTAL RELAXATION THERAPIES

The human brain is an integral part of the human body, controlling the body's basic functions when asleep or awake. To some extent, any individual can exert conscious control over the body's vital signs: the heart rate, for example, can be speeded up by breathing rapidly. The brain also controls the release of stress hormones, which activate the natural "fight-or-flight" response. Chemicals in the brain also react to various stimuli to induce emotional states such as excitement, sadness, or fright. A person's physical health can be subject to simple hope and expectation: In the placebo effect, for example, a pill containing no medication whatsoever, when given to an individual told of its effectiveness, actually can affect the biochemical makeup of the body and relieve symptoms of an illness.

Mental relaxation therapies rely on this intimate mind/body connection. These techniques work through the use of mental imagery and verbal suggestion to relieve stress. When the therapy is complex, a physician or guide can serve as an instructor. Several of these therapies are simple enough to be practiced alone in the comfort of a familiar room.

Hypnosis

The practice of hypnosis seeks to create a deeply relaxed physical and mental state known as a hypnotic trance. This allows an individual to act on suggestions made by the hypnotist. Although a person in a hypnotic trance remains aware and awake, the suggestions are received without the normal "screening" functions of the conscious mind. There is no judgment or opinion formed about the suggestion. The person under hypnosis is not distracted by conditions in the environment or by inner emotions and perceptions, shyness, or anxiety.

A hypnosis patient might see a practitioner for an hour or a half hour, once a week, in a private office. In group hypnosis, several people gather together for a common treatment of physical or mental symptoms. To place an individual under a hypnotic trance, a hypnotist asks the individual to relax in a seated position, then focus on an object placed directly in the person's line of sight. Eventually, while keeping this focus and under instructions to clear the mind and relax, the eyes will close and usually the actual hypnosis session can begin.

To combat stress, a direct hypnotic suggestion can be made. The suggestion is meant to change one's perception of events. The suggestion is framed as if it comes directly from the person under hypnosis. A recent negative event such as an argument or confrontation can be dismissed with the suggestion that "this doesn't bother me too much." A posthypnotic suggestion can also help to alter behavior and perception in the future, after the hypnotic trance is finished. For example, "I will feel more relaxed at work" or "I will not feel shy when meeting new people."

Hypnosis has been used in cases of acute anxiety. It also has helped people overcome insomnia, eating disorders, and disabling phobias such as the fear of flying or the fear of water. In the course of some psychotherapy, hypnosis is sometimes used to make suggestions to the patient that help him or her overcome the effects of stress on the body and mind.

Q & A

Question: Can a hypnotist make me do anything?

Answer: Hypnosis works through the power of suggestion, which in a hypnotic trance goes directly to the *subconscious.* However, a person under hypnosis remains in control of his or her actions. He or she will not go into a hypnotic trance without wanting to do so. Once in the trance, a person remains conscious of his or her surroundings and will refuse to do anything contrary to his physical and emotional well-being.

Visualization

The connection between the conscious mind and the physical state of the body is made directly with visualization, or imagery. Under guidance, a person closes the eyes and imagines a peaceful, relaxing scene, either created on one's own or suggested by someone else. These visualizations are used to directly confront stressful ideas or situations and help the patient associate a more relaxed state of mind with whatever that situation may be.

Meditation

Rather than placing a specific image in mind, meditation seeks to empty the mind of any outside sensation and turn thoughts inward. In a meditation session, a person sits quietly, alone, in a room free of distraction. A single sound—a mantra—is repeated steadily while breathing comes under control. By concentrating on the mantra, the meditator is able to temporarily silence the inner voice that is constantly making judgments, issuing directions, and worrying about the future. In certain meditative states, a person can reach a state of heightened awareness in which he or she perceives the environment but remains completely detached from those surroundings.

Meditation is a method for achieving a state of complete mental relaxation, lowering stress, and becoming more detached while remaining acutely aware of the outside world. Effective meditation also has physical effects, slowing the body's metabolism and steadying the heart rate and breathing. Those who spend a few minutes every day meditating report a decrease in the general feeling of anxiety when confronted by stressful demands, the need to make decisions, and a stream of worrying "self-talk."

Biofeedback

In biofeedback therapy, a patient or doctor monitors the physical results of a mental or physical process. Biofeedback uses an array of instruments that measure changes in skin temperature, muscle tension, pulse, blood pressure, and brain waves. By using these instruments, a person practicing a relaxation technique can see immediate results in the changes in his or her own vital signs.

Biofeedback therapy was once a highly specialized medical niche, a subject of experimentation in clinical laboratories. This research showed that the **autonomic nervous system,** which controls the automatic functions of the body, can be placed under voluntary control—not just by humans, but by any conscious animal. Recently, biofeedback instruments have become available to anyone.

There are a variety of biofeedback monitors, each with a specialized use. An electromyelograph (EMG) measures muscle tension. A person can use an EMG to control this tension and ease the pain of headaches or backaches. In the same manner, a thermistor, which measures skin temperature, can be useful. A drop in skin temperature, caused by constriction of the vessels carrying blood to the extremities, indicates a stress response. A fairly reliable relaxation therapy, biofeedback can help people recognize and overcome stress.

PHYSICAL RELAXATION THERAPIES

Muscular tension is one of the most common reactions to stress. Certain kinds of stress seem to cause certain muscles to respond in this way. Neck muscles, for example, often grow stiff in a person unable to express emotion, as the face and head are purposefully kept rigid. Bouts of anger often bring muscle pain in the chest and abdomen. When muscles tense, blood circulation is hindered and lactic acid and other waste products build up in the affected tissue. The result is a sense of fatigue and restlessness that often accompanies a stressful episode.

Physical exercise is one of the most effective ways to release muscle tension and stress. There are several specialized methods of muscle relaxation that have the same effect. These methods are designed to quiet the mind as they work the body. They are designed to subdue the mild, continuous stress response that occurs throughout a busy day.

Progressive Muscle Relaxation

The technique of progressive muscle relaxation, also known as Jacobson relaxation, can be practiced alone, without a doctor's guidance. The person finds a quiet room free of distractions and sits comfortably. Moving around the body, he or she tenses groups of muscles such as those in the lower leg, holding the tension for 15 seconds, then letting it go while breathing out. One variation on progressive relaxation is the Mitchell method, in which parts of the body assume relaxed positions that are naturally different from those associated with tension and stress. The Mitchell method is often taught in combination with deep breathing exercises, which focus on a slow and rhythmic intake of breath from the abdomen, rather than from the upper chest.

Autogenic Training

This method directs a person to focus on specific sensations in the body, such as warmth, coolness, or heaviness in the hands or arms. By this method, an individual becomes more aware of the physical effects of stress and learns to cope with them directly, without guidance.

Autogenic training is a form of self-hypnosis. The person begins by consciously relaxing any parts of the body that feel tense. Then he or she repeats a familiar series of messages, such as:

My left arm is heavy.

Both arms are heavy.

My right leg is heavy.

My left leg is heavy.

Both legs are heavy.

My neck and shoulders are heavy.

I am at peace.

My right arm is warm.

My left arm is warm.

My right leg is warm.

My left leg is warm.

My neck and shoulders are warm.

I am at peace.

The body parts follow the conscious instructions, and gradually physical sensations follow the guidance of the words. With practice, the autogenic "scripts" become more familiar and repeat without any mental effort. Autogenic sessions can end with a physical relaxation therapy or a series of affirmations, in which the person repeats positive messages about the results.

Yoga

Yoga has become one of the most popular methods of physical exercise and stress reduction. Yoga sessions take place under the guidance of a trained instructor. During the course of a one- or two-hour yoga session, participants assume a series of postures intended to stretch, strengthen, and balance the body. The session usually ends with a short period of meditation or **guided imagery**. This allows the body to cool down after a strenuous workout and the mind to focus inward.

Of the several different schools of yoga, some are relatively easy, while some are more advanced and difficult. Bikram yoga is designed to relax and limber up the muscles, then sweat out physical stress. Kripalu yoga is a more mentally focused form of yoga, in which the instructor guides a student through a series of easy postures and meditation.

Yoga helps many people to set aside normal, everyday stresses such as overwork, family troubles, arguments with friends, or confrontations with strangers. The meditative aspect of a yoga class helps students to achieve a more detached and calm attitude to their social environments.

Brief Methods

Many people follow a relaxation therapy of their own. They develop a daily routine, either in the morning or evening, of those practices they find most effective in achieving balance. There are also unstructured methods of temporary or brief relaxation, which can be practiced at any time of the day without a schedule or routine. These include steady, paced breathing, done for a few minutes while the eyes are closed and the body relaxed. The person draws in breath from the abdomen, holds it for up to five seconds, then slowly lets it out.

DID YOU KNOW?

The 26 Postures of Bikram Yoga

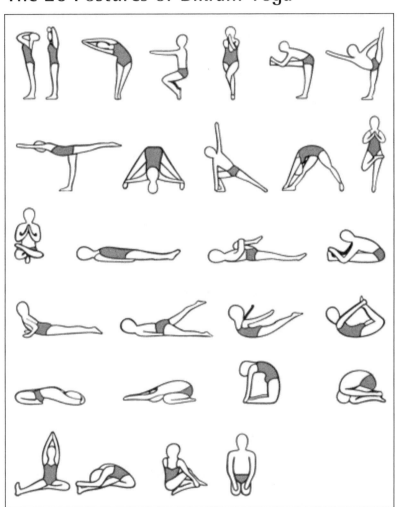

In Bikram yoga, students follow a series of 26 asanas or postures while working in a room heated to 105 degrees Fahrenheit.

Source: http://www.indianabikram.com/wpcontent/uploads/postures.jpg

Many people face common situations with a sense of anxiety. An elevator ride, for example, can prompt a stress response in people with a fear of enclosed spaces. A meeting with a teacher, a dentist's appointment, or any impending confrontation can also lead to a "fight-or-flight" reaction, the release of stress hormones, and negative physical and mental responses.

As long as physical action is not needed, a person facing an immediate stressful situation can respond with a series of deep breaths, repeating a simple word or syllable in a short meditation. Deep focus on a simple object such as a picture or a flower can also calm the stress response and help to clear the mind of anxious self-talk.

See also: Meditation; Stress Management Techniques; Treatment

FURTHER READING

Casey, Aggie, and Herbert Benson. *Mind Your Heart: A Mind/Body Approach to Stress Management, Exercise, and Nutrition for Heart Health.* New York: Free Press, 2004.

Donaghy, Marie, Rosemary A. Payne, and Keith Bellamy. *Relaxation Techniques: A Practical Guide for the Health Care Professional.* Edinburgh, U.K.: Churchill Livingstone, 2005.

McCall, Timothy. *Yoga as Medicine: The Yogic Prescription for Health and Healing.* New York: Bantam, 2007.

Sharples, Bob. *Meditation and Relaxation in Plain English.* Boston: Wisdom Publications, 2006.

■ SLEEP AND STRESS

A period of rest for the mind and body, the deprivation of which will impair memory, brain function, and reflexes. Sleep is a natural function of all animals, including humans. A period of sleep is essential to the proper functioning of the body and the brain. Depriving yourself of sleep results in memory loss, impaired coordination, headaches, nausea, rising blood pressure, and in severe cases hallucinations and psychosis.

High stress levels affect a person's ability to sleep. In turn, a lack of sleep contributes to high stress. Breaking the cycle of stress and sleeplessness is crucial to overcoming the physical and mental harm that occurs in a stressful lifestyle.

WHAT IS SLEEP?

While sleeping, the brain enters a period of unconsciousness. A sleeping person no longer reacts to most outside stimuli such as lights and noises and loses voluntary control of the muscles. Rapid-eye movement (REM) takes place during certain periods of sleep; non-REM sleep is more common in the earlier stages. Scientists have divided non-REM sleep into several stages, which take place over cycles of about 90 minutes. The deepest sleep takes place earlier in the sleeping period, while lighter REM sleep periods are more common toward the end of the cycle. If deprived of sleep for long periods of time, people will grow seriously impaired. They will lose the ability to remember and calculate, suffer headaches and fatigue, and even gain weight (as appetite increases and the digestive system slows down).

Scientists study sleep by examining brain waves on an electroencephalograph, or EEG. Each stage of sleep brings a certain brain-wave frequency, with the deepest stage characterized by slow "delta" waves. At this stage, it is most difficult for a sleeping person to wake up. If awakened, he or she will take a longer period of time to recover conscious mental abilities. If deprived of slow-wave sleep, then returned to normal sleep, the body will enter longer and more frequent periods of deep sleep until the deficit is made up.

Young people experience more deep sleep than adults, and the elderly get the least amount of sleep per night. Even when allowed to fall asleep and wake up normally, some older people will catch only short periods of deep sleep, or none at all. Warmer body temperature, physical exercise, and a high-carbohydrate diet all increase the amount of deep sleep a person gets.

Q & A

Question: How much sleep do I need?

Answer: Although eight hours is the traditional amount of sleep that adults should get, according to many scientific studies, nine or 10 hours is necessary for teenagers. Several studies have found that adults who sleep six to seven hours a night have longer life expectancy. However, there's just one catch: They must wake up naturally, rather than using an alarm clock.

STRESS HORMONES AND SLEEP

Stress hormones released by the endocrine system increase wakefulness, as the body prepares for "fight or flight." However, an excess of stress hormones in the bloodstream can also make it difficult to sleep.

The Sleepless Society

For many people, the contemporary world is a scene of constant, low-level stress. Worries over health, money, school, and family cause a state of perpetual anxiety and bring about the natural reaction of the body to a problem: the release of adrenaline, cortisol, and other hormones meant for sudden physical activity. This is the reason behind what some researchers have called an epidemic of insomnia and sleep deprivation.

Sleep Deprivation

According to many surveys, as much as half of the population of the United States is getting six hours or less of sleep every night, an amount that most researchers believe is not enough to rest the mind and body. Sleep deprivation is often intentional: People push back optional bedtimes to complete work or study and wake up earlier to make it on time to an office or school.

Wakefulness

Wakefulness at night is another symptom of stressful living. A study conducted by researchers of the Pennsylvania State University College of Medicine found this problem growing in middle-aged men. The study found that as men age they become more sensitive to corticotrophin-releasing hormone, or CRH, a hormone that brings about the release of cortisol. This in turn hinders their ability to sleep normally.

Insomnia

In society as a whole, insomnia (the inability to fall or stay asleep) is becoming a common problem. There are many possible reasons for a case of insomnia, which at its worst can deprive a person of sleep for several days running. Scientists have made one important connection in finding that insomniacs release more cortisol than those who enjoy normal sleep. High levels of stress bring about high levels of cortisol, which in turn affect the brain's ability to temporarily shut down at night.

Social and environmental factors are at work as well. For many people, work no longer ends at quitting time. Instead, the work and the stress that comes with it are brought home. This is true for students

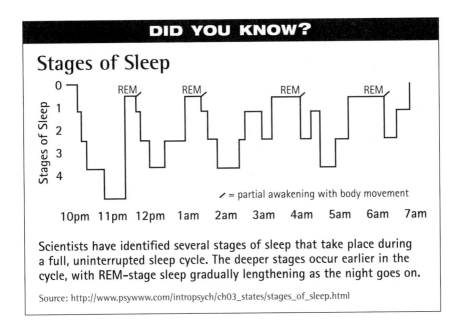

DID YOU KNOW?

Stages of Sleep

↗ = partial awakening with body movement

Scientists have identified several stages of sleep that take place during a full, uninterrupted sleep cycle. The deeper stages occur earlier in the cycle, with REM-stage sleep gradually lengthening as the night goes on.

Source: http://www.psywww.com/intropsych/ch03_states/stages_of_sleep.html

with heavy homework loads. For better sleep, it is a good idea to take care of homework in the late afternoon or early evening.

"All-Nighters"

When faced with a presentation or an exam, many people also will make the unwise decision to work past their normal sleep time. This interrupts a natural circadian rhythm of sleep and wakefulness that is regulated by the release of hormones in the body. When sleep begins later than normal, or when an "all-nighter" is pulled in preparation for the next day's event, the morning brings grogginess, irritability, and impaired mental function. Getting the usual sleep is a much better idea, as an unconscious mind can process problems about as well as a wakeful one. Realizing this, many people will pose a difficult problem to themselves at night, consider all of the elements necessary to solve that problem, then get a full night's sleep. Often, the result in the morning is a clear and easy solution.

Q & A

Question: Because I didn't sleep well, should I just drink a lot of coffee?

Answer: Coffee contains caffeine, a stimulant that goes to work on your nervous system within 15 minutes of your first sip. It blocks the production of sleep-producing hormones and increases the production of adrenaline, the necessary "fight-or-flight" hormone that goes to work when you face a stressful situation.

According to a recent poll, 43 percent of Americans reported they were "very likely" to drink coffee during the day if they felt sleepy. Coffee cannot replace sleep, however, and too much coffee can make you anxious, irritable, and nervous. Coffee in large doses can increase the heart rate, cause digestive problems, and make it hard to fall asleep at night. Experts recommend not drinking any coffee, or ingesting other forms of caffeine, later than six hours before bedtime.

SOLVING THE SLEEP/STRESS PROBLEM

Doctors advise sleep-deprived patients of several ways to overcome their inability to get a good night's rest. Relaxation techniques such as meditation, yoga, and autogenic training can help people forget, temporarily, the problems and worries that have arisen during a stressful day. Walking or light exercise in the evening can help as well. Studies also have found that people who regularly engage their minds with mental exercises, games, and hobbies also have a better capacity for restful sleep.

The challenges of a tough academic program or a job can stimulate a person to greater effort, but striving also can lead to higher levels of stress and sleeplessness. Psychologists often advise sleep-deprived patients to reconsider their priorities in life and think about the trade-off between more money in a better, more stressful job, for example, and physical and mental health. A lack of sleep may not indicate just a higher concentration of stress hormones; it may also be a gauge of an individual's taking on more responsibility than he or she is designed or prepared to handle.

Stress and Stimulants

Sleep experts advise avoiding stressful situations during the evening, if possible. It is also not a good idea to drink coffee or other stimulants such as sugary soft drinks or energy drinks after the mid-afternoon. Heavy alcohol use can disrupt normal sleep patterns as well. Although it seems one way to slow the body down, watching television from the comfort of a couch is not the ideal way to prepare for sleep, as some shows in themselves can trigger stress and anxiety.

Napping

Naps are another effective way to combat sleeplessness and stress. The body begins to slow down after eight hours of wakefulness. At this time, a nap of 20 to 30 minutes can restore energy and help the body overcome the effects of stress earlier in the day. Going through an entire single natural sleep cycle, then waking up, will bring about a higher state of alertness for the balance of the day. Longer naps are not advised, as a stage of deep sleep that might begin makes it more difficult both to wake up and then to fall asleep again at night.

Sleeping Environment

Finally, one of the best ways to manage sleep is to control the sleeping environment. One's bedroom should be free of computers, televisions, and work activities. It should be kept at a comfortable temperature, without distracting clutter such as scattered clothes, books, and papers. The bed should be neither too big nor too small, and with a mattress neither very hard nor too soft. A sleeping environment should also be quiet and not a place for dealing with serious, stressful matters that will bring additional anxiety.

See also: Stress Management Techniques; Treatment

FURTHER READING

Dement, William C. *The Promise of Sleep: A Pioneer in Sleep Medicine Explores the Vital Connection Between Health, Happiness, and a Good Night's Sleep.* New York: Dell, 2000.

Epstein, Lawrence, and Steven Mardon. *The Harvard Medical School Guide to a Good Night's Sleep.* New York: McGraw-Hill, 2006.

Schenck, Carlos H. *Sleep: A Groundbreaking Guide to the Mysteries, the Problems, and the Solutions.* New York: Avery, 2008.

▣ STRESS AND THE ENVIRONMENT

Physical and psychological responses to one's physical surroundings. Factors such as crowding or unfamiliarity can make a stressful situation more difficult to control or resolve. An ongoing lack of control over environmental conditions can also lead to a case of chronic mental or physical stress.

Fact Or Fiction?

A building can make you sick.

The Facts: Serious illnesses can be caused by environmental hazards found in some buildings and homes. These hazards can include the use of **toxic** construction or maintenance materials; mold or mildew caused by a poor ventilation system; the creation of ozone by electronic equipment and copiers; the presence of artificial dyes and fragrances; smoking; or the presence of asbestos. When many people in a workplace suddenly report symptoms of fatigue, headaches, skin irritations, and breathing problems, a building itself can be diagnosed with "sick building syndrome." These types of environmental hazards are the result of human activity.

WORKPLACES

Poor conditions in an office or school can easily create stress. Classrooms, for example, can be crowded and noisy places, especially when teachers have problems keeping students quiet and attentive. This makes it difficult for students to concentrate on lessons, take tests, or learn. According to a survey by the American Association of School Administrators, 44 percent of all school districts increased their average class size for the school year 2009–10. In Los Angeles, for example, the average class size for junior and senior high school students was 43. There is little to be done about crowded classes, however, when the economy struggles and school budgets are cut.

Crowded classrooms contribute to clutter and disorganization. They also tend to create more interruptions, accidents, and noise. This makes it more difficult for people to accomplish tasks, placing more stress on everyone involved: students, supervisors, and teachers. A sense of personal disorganization contributes to the inability to get work done. Messy rooms lead to lost belongings, arguments, and a sense of apathy about one's physical surroundings. All these factors are very common **stressors.**

A stress-inducing environment may also await those leaving the workplace or school. Increasingly crowded streets result in traffic jams, noise, and air pollution, causing people to react with anger and frustration. A 2007 "Urban Mobility Report" by the Texas Transportation Institute found that commuting nationwide wasted 2.9 billion gallons of fuel and 4.2 billion work hours, equivalent to 105 million weeks of vacation.

Heavy commuting arose in the years after World War II, when cities expanded into suburban metropolitan areas, and a vast network of freeways was designed to allow drivers to quickly motor from point to point. Suburbs grew as families sought out the serenity and security of homes away from noisy inner cities. One result was the stressful work or school commute, which wastes an increasing amount of time for society as a whole.

PERSONAL ENVIRONMENTS

Lack of physical comfort is another aspect of one's surroundings that can be a source of stress. Badly designed furniture, poor lighting, extreme heat, extreme cold, and a lack of air circulation all contribute to physical stress. Other sources of discomfort include sitting for long periods in an office or classroom chair, thereby putting a strain on the back, and hunching over a computer keyboard, which creates neck strain, eyestrain, and carpal tunnel syndrome (an inflammation of ligaments in the wrist).

Cubicle Stress

The modern workplace is not a place for physical exercise or even short periods of calm and relaxation. Many offices have an open-plan design, with workers assigned to small cubicles, separated by dividers at eye level, in a single large room. While cubicles have no doors or ceilings, they also drastically limit the field of vision.

This design imposes both isolation and a lack of privacy. Although they may be able to work alone in a semi-private space, cubicle workers are also subject to constant noise and interruptions. A study done by Dr. Vinesh Oommen, a researcher at Queensland University of Technology in Brisbane, Australia, found that 90 percent of open-plan offices led to more negative consequences, including higher levels of stress, conflict, and staff turnover, compared to small, private offices.

Environmental stress forces the body to seek adjustments: a change in position or posture, better light or air, and less noisy surroundings. When these adjustments prove difficult or impossible to make, a stress reaction begins; the sense of building frustration leads to the release of **stress hormones** into the bloodstream, prompting a "fight-or-flight" reaction. A chronic stress reaction that does not resolve leads to a higher level of these hormones, which can bring about a wide range of negative physical responses: headaches, high blood pressure, sleeplessness, digestive problems, anxiety, and depression.

Air Quality

One of the most common, and serious, threats to the physical environment, and therefore a source of stress, is poor air quality. Dust and pollutants circulate freely if ventilation is poor. Many modern homes and offices often have windows that seal the interior against fresh air. The problem is worse in warm-weather regions that rely on air conditioning to provide comfort on hot days. If air filters are old or in poor condition, air will not circulate and the pollution levels rise from carpet, furniture, chemicals, and office equipment. Where smoking is allowed, people are also subject to higher levels of air pollution. The result is more physical stress in the form of headaches, fatigue, allergic reactions, and illness.

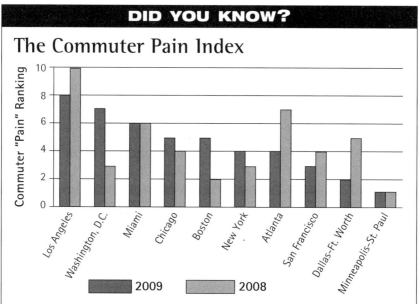

DID YOU KNOW?

The Commuter Pain Index

Created by the IBM corporation, this chart ranks the emotional and economic costs of commuting in 10 metropolitan areas on a scale of 1 to 10. The 10 aspects of commuting included in the index are commuting time, time stuck in traffic, and value of time; and the agreement of people responding to the survey that: traffic has gotten worse, start-stop traffic is a problem, driving causes stress, driving causes anger, traffic affects work, traffic gets so bad that driving stopped, and "decided not to make trip due to traffic."

Source: IBM Commuter Pain Study Chart at http://www-03.ibm.com/press/us/en/photo/28321.wss

One common solution to alleviate poor air quality is to install plants in a closed room. When properly cared for, plants provide oxygen, reduce carbon dioxide levels, and help to humidify dry air.

Lighting

Poorly lit classrooms or work areas also put stress on students and employees. Artificial light, light that is too dim, or light that is too bright can bring about a stress reaction.

A lack of natural light from windows hinders the body in the functioning of circadian rhythms, which control sleep and wakefulness. This problem can become acute in the winter, when days are shorter and periods of natural light are brief. Workers who arrive and leave their offices in darkness are subject to depression, weight gain (overeating is a common response to anxiety or depression), an "afternoon slump" in which energy is at a minimum, and a loss of the ability to concentrate. This reaction is called Seasonal Affective Disorder, or SAD, and sometimes can be treated with the use of special lamps that imitate the natural light of the sun.

Color

Another environmental factor affecting mood and stress is color. People have common associations with certain colors, including, for example, red (angry, emotional); green (calm); and black (depressive). One of these colors on a wall, floor, or even in the furniture one uses can evoke that emotional reaction. This is one possible explanation as to why rooms for actors and musicians preparing to go onstage are "green rooms," and why casinos have a lot of gilded, glittering surfaces, causing an unconscious association with money and success.

DE-STRESSING THE ENVIRONMENT

One's physical surroundings then can cause negative physical or psychological reactions as well as make it more difficult to deal with any acute stresses or emergencies that arise. To avoid stress caused by the environment, there are several actions one can take:

- Whenever you study or work, maintain the room in a neat, clean, and organized fashion. Get rid of unused or unnecessary objects. Organize your desk or workspace at the end of every day.

- Ensure that you have privacy and quiet when needed but that you can also interact with others freely.

- Use furniture that is comfortable and places minimal stress on the body.
- Ensure adequate light and try to have as much natural light available as possible.
- Avoid **toxic** air by avoiding smoking, changing air filters, making sure ventilation equipment is working properly, and allowing in natural air from time to time.
- If a daily commute is causing high stress, consider a more convenient job or school, or, if possible, move to a home closer to your destination.
- Solve the problem of high noise levels by using screens, carpets, or plants that can help absorb sound.

See also: Emotional Stress; Stress and the Workplace; Types of Stress

FURTHER READING
Hutchings, Patricia J. *Managing Workplace Chaos: Workplace Solutions for Managing Information, Paper, Time, and Stress.* New York: AMACOM Books, 2002.
Lim, Jess T. Y. *Feng Shui for Business and Office.* Toronto, Canada: Warwick, 2003.

■ STRESS AND THE FAMILY

Sources of conflict as they may exist in the traditional, extended, blended, alternative, and/or racially mixed family. A common view holds the home and family as a source of stability and support. In this perception, the family is an oasis, where different individuals pull together to meet outside challenges. However, the perception is not always the reality; one of the most significant sources of emotional stress, for any gender or age, is the family.

Stress in the family typically arises from the many demands placed on its members and the inability of the members of the household to work together to meet its needs. Often, family stress comes from an important change such as a move to a new home, children entering or leaving school, or parents going through a separation or divorce. School and work pressures add to the stress level. Also, as children develop into adolescents and then adults, conflict with parents can be almost constant.

FINANCIAL WORRIES

Economic problems also place stress on the family. According to a study by Valerie Adrian and Stephanie Coontz for the Council on Contemporary Families, the most important sources of family stress are job losses, rising gas prices, and a new phenomenon known as "residential insecurity," the stress that arises from being unable to afford a mortgage or rent payment.

FAMILY ARGUMENTS

A family under heavy stress can turn a household into a battle zone, where arguments are constant and emotions run high. The feeling of losing control, as well as feeling trapped in an unpleasant situation, can cause every family member to react to **stressors** with negative behavior.

Family stress affects not just one individual but the entire household. When an illness, personal conflict, or other stressor affects one member, the other family members experience their own difficulty in facing this trouble and dealing with it, sometimes every day.

Signs and symptoms

Families may experience one or several signs of stress. These include a sense of urgency and a lack of time to accomplish anything, or to spend together. Individuals may experience a sense of frustration and an inability to relax. Bickering and arguing can become more frequent and begin to invade even ordinary conversation about insignificant problems. Daily pleasures such as eating meals together become rushed and hectic or silent and unpleasant. Individual members may escape to their rooms, to the workplace, or to a group of friends.

LIFE EVENTS

All families go through transitions or important life events. Not necessarily negative, these events can include the birth of a new member or graduation from high school. However, all life events demand some adapting. Family members have to adjust their schedules, their living arrangements, or their place in the family hierarchy. Overnight, for example, an only child can become an older sibling, who must share the attention of parents. This is a difficult transition that can cause reactions from everyone in the home.

A sudden life event can complicate even the most peaceful family situation and raise the stress level. If one of the household's wage earners unexpectedly loses a job, the family must adjust to several stressors at once: financial problems, the emotional stress of unemployment, the need to job search, or a forced move out of a home. An accident in the home, a sudden illness, a runaway teen, even a surprise visit from relatives can all envelop families in chronic stress.

CHRONIC STRESSORS

The ongoing, everyday habits of a family can be experienced differently by different members of the family. Parents following a busy daily schedule must arrange for transportation, plan school events, prepare meals, supervise homework, and do the shopping. They must clean and maintain the home, work outside the home to earn money, and make plans for holidays and vacations.

Children and teenagers, on the other hand, on a daily basis must attend school, take part in extracurricular activities, finish homework, help with household chores, and keep their rooms tidy. The expectations of parents can clash with their children's needs and desires, which were more readily met when they were younger. When repeated every day, simple chores can become stress-inducing burdens, bringing on a case of burnout.

Children can also place a heavy burden of stress on parents. As the child grows into a toddler, the demand for material goods increases. Studies have linked exposure to television and advertising to children's demand for toys and objects. Eventually, these demands work. The tried-and-true technique of nagging, for example, resulted in 40 percent of all visits to Chuck E. Cheese and other childhood entertainment venues and one-third of all visits to fast-food restaurants.

The chronic everyday stress affects men and women differently. A study by Neala S. Schwartzberg and Rita Scher Dytell, published in the *Journal of Occupational Health Psychology*, found that for parents who both earn income, time pressure was less stressful than the pressure of having to fulfill different roles: breadwinner and caregiver. The researchers also found that for both mothers and fathers, self-esteem and a sense of accomplishment came more from work, while emotional balance and well-being came from the home. For fathers, stress came more from a lack of support from their spouses and a loss of importance in the home. For mothers, stress came from a sense of isolation, of heavier home responsibilities, and a lack of help with household chores.

Fact Or Fiction?

Stress decreases as the school year ends.

The Facts: Stress *increases* at the end of the school year. Final exams make the last week a time of worry over graduation and grades. The uncertainty of summer jobs and activities causes anxiety. The temporary loss of classmate friends can depress students. Summer vacation also brings the prospect of several weeks of boredom and a lot more time at home with siblings and parents—not a relaxing idea for many teenagers.

STRESS EXPERIENCE

The perception of stressors plays a crucial role in a family's reaction to stress. Some families have more experience than others at dealing with sudden life events. Military families, for example, move often from one assigned location to the next—and are more experienced and capable of dealing with the stress of a move. To help cope with this kind of stress, family members might see such a transition as an opportunity rather than a difficulty.

The outlook of individual family members also plays a part. Some people are simply wired for stress—they are type A personalities who thrive on difficult challenges and get accustomed to a higher stress level. Type A behavior is learned; some parents will pass it on with the goals and expectations they set for children, while others will allow more freedom and a different outlook on life and work. When family members have different reactions to stress, however, the entire household can find it more difficult to cooperate in the face of an important change.

Each family uses different resources to cope with stress. The key resource is the ability to communicate with one another. Families with a strong hierarchy find it easier to reach decisions. Those with a large network of friends, relatives, and close neighbors, as well as roots in the community where they live, also are better prepared.

CRISIS AND BREAKDOWN

A serious and threatening event such as a car accident or fire can throw a family into an emergency situation. One of the members may fall into addiction, come down with a life-threatening illness, or suffer expulsion from school. A case of acute stress arises that affects every member. Physical effects can appear in individuals, arising from the stress reaction that all members are experiencing. Families that are close and that have been through such an emergency before might cope and survive. Families with loose ties have a more difficult time.

In modern society, the trend is toward families with looser ties and less common experience. Parents and children follow their own careers, which place heavy demands on their time and attention. The family becomes a collection of individuals, often living under the same roof but sharing fewer activities and interests. When parents spend less time with children, each member becomes more isolated, less able to deal with sudden or chronic problems. This can magnify the effect of stress on an individual member.

Domestic Violence

Severe family stress can lead to a case of domestic violence, which can take several forms. In an abusive or violent relationship, coercion and threats are used to gain control over someone's life or actions. Violent behavior can steadily escalate, from threats to expressions of anger such as throwing or destroying objects, displaying weapons, or abusing pets or favorite objects. Retaliation raises the violence level, so that angry words lead to physical abuse and assaults.

More subtle is emotional abuse, which can leave a lasting, unseen psychological mark on the victim. This takes the form of putdowns, name-calling, and making someone feel guilty or humiliated over their past mistakes or thwarted ambitions. Parents can also subject their children to the stress of isolation: forcing them into their rooms, banning friends from the house, and forbidding any use of the phone or computer. According to the National Coalition against Domestic Violence (NCADV), the victims of emotional and physical abuse are mostly women. In a 2007 statistical survey, the NCADV found that one in every four women will experience domestic violence in their lifetimes; 1.3 million women are subject to a physical assault by a domestic partner each year; and 85 percent of domestic violence victims are women.

Child Abuse and Neglect

Another upshot of extreme stress in the family can be a case of child abuse or neglect. Financial, emotional, or other forms of stress can lead to a neglect of a child's need for food, shelter, clothing, and basic comforts. Children may be blamed for increasing the family's financial burdens or causing divisions between the parents and with other siblings. Since most children don't have the resources to act on their own or prevent acts of abuse, many cases are never reported.

According to the U.S. Department of Health and Human Services, child abuse results when "any recent act or failure to act on the part of a parent or caretaker which results in death, serious physical or emotional harm, sexual abuse or exploitation; or an act or failure to act which presents an imminent risk of serious harm." In 2007, the agency estimated that 794,000 children were the victims of maltreatment, a rate of 10.6 per 1,000 children. In the same period, more than 3.5 million cases of abuse or neglect were investigated by state child protection services.

Separation and Divorce

In households where parents are unable to overcome their differences, separation or divorce can result, bringing the nuclear family to an end and subjecting the members of the family to relocation, isolation, loneliness, anxiety, and depression. Chronic stress on families is a major cause of high divorce rates in Europe and the United States. A study published by the *Journal of Social and Personal Relationships* surveyed more than 600 divorced couples and found that these couples saw lack of communication and the inability to cope with or solve problems as more important than stress in breaking their relationships. But the study also found that as they build up, trivial everyday stressors were key reasons for the final decision to go through a divorce.

In the United States, the number of divorces has been gradually declining for several years, as has the number of marriages. In 2008, there were 2,162,000 marriages, about 7.1 per 1,000 total population. The divorce rate stood at 3.5 per 1,000. As a percentage of marriages, divorces were just below 50 percent, a rate that has been holding steady for several decades.

TEENS SPEAK

A Day in the Life

I'm not sure if I'm in a normal family. We spend most of the time arguing. It starts when I get up in the morning. My parents start giving instructions even before they say good morning. They also give me some advice and offer a few criticisms. I get the feeling that I'm in the army. Maybe the army would be a nice break.

When I get home, the stress just keeps on. My sister is crying about something, and I'm supposed to figure out what it is and then solve her problem. When she feels better, she goes to her room and slams the door. My mom says let her have some privacy. If I do the same, then I'm being antisocial.

Dinner is the highlight. We talk about things I'm supposed to get done. Do this, do that. If I don't do them, then bad things will happen. Everyone will suffer if I go back to my old habits and get lazy again. For me, it's not laziness, it's just down time. I need to get away once in a while. In fact, I need to get away as often as possible.

Things get a little better on Friday night, but not much. That's family night. We go out to a restaurant or a movie. Sometimes we keep on arguing, but usually we talk things over. Everyone gets to share their problem, whatever it is. When that happens, and we agree on a few things, the whole weekend seems to go a little better.

COPING

Many families cope with stress by drawing on quality time. This is a planned opportunity for shared experience, held in the home or outside the home. Quality time, in theory, builds communication among the members of a family. A sense of togetherness, even if only temporary, helps the family cope with chronic stress or unexpected problems.

Some of the best quality time, ironically, involves work. This includes physical work: cleaning, sweeping, repairing, and maintaining the home. Cooperating in such chores improves communication, allows for stress-defeating exercise, and improves the house's condition, which by itself can become a source of chronic family stress.

Sharing meals is another approach to achieving quality time. At one time, it was customary for families to share a dinner at the same time each day, and with each member present. This was the time for planning and problem solving. Modern families under time pressure and with conflicting schedules can find it difficult to arrange traditional evening meals. Many find it easier to meet for breakfast instead. Counselors often advise families under pressure to schedule at least one meal a day together.

Communication

To cope with stress, open discussion is also key. An individual dealing with a stressor will eventually have an effect on other members. At first, the other members may not see the problem as important. If the stress continues, then the individual experiencing it may begin to feel more isolated within the family or start to blame the other members for doing nothing to help. He or she may also be the target of blame: By reacting to a stressful situation, the entire family is faced with a new problem.

Privacy

While communication is useful, a respect for privacy also helps a family deal with stress. Some personal problems are difficult to share. If a daughter is dealing with a suddenly hostile friend, she may need to talk it out with a parent but would rather not have siblings know anything about it. She will share the issue only in confidence; if the confidence is broken, trust will dwindle away, and the family will find it harder to solve a case of acute stress in the future.

The flip side of a respect for privacy is receptivity to openness, especially when making critical decisions. Parents facing marital troubles often keep their problems secret. Eventually, however, if the problem begins to threaten the survival of the family, then one or both parents must begin to share the source of stress with children.

Families that have accustomed themselves to stress can better deal with more stress. They tend to have more time together, communicate openly, and are more flexible and less demanding of one another. They also become familiar with useful strategies for coping: becoming realistic about the amount of work each member can get done, making lists and prioritizing activities, and making time to relax.

See also: Emotional Stress; Holiday Stress; Types of Stress

FURTHER READING
Boss, Pauline, ed. *Family Stress: Classic and Contemporary Readings.* Newbury Park, Calif.: Sage Publications, 2002.
Cassella-Kapusinski, *Now What Do I Do? A Guide to Helping Teenagers with Their Parents' Separation and Divorce.* Skokie, Ill.: ACTA Publications, 2006.
LeBey, Barbara. *Family Estrangements: How They Begin, How to Mend Them, How to Cope with Them.* New York: Bantam Books, 2003.

■ STRESS AND THE HEART

The way we react to certain events and the impact of these reactions on the heart. The heart is a muscle about the size of a fist. Its function is simple: to circulate blood through the body. It beats on average about 70 times per minute, moving blood from the two upper chambers (the atria) through the two lower chambers (the ventricles), and then through arteries to the rest of the body.

HEART DISEASE

Heart, or cardiovascular, disease is the leading cause of death in the United States. Without proper heart function, the health of the body will decline. A heart attack—a break in the supply of blood to the heart—can result in damage to the circulatory system, or death. Hypertension, or high blood pressure, can also damage the heart. Stress is an important cause of hypertension.

Many individuals suffer from coronary artery disease, in which a blockage forms in the arteries and the heart gradually loses its ability to move blood through the body. Symptoms of coronary artery disease are chest pain, fatigue, dizziness, and **arrhythmia:** an irregular heart beat. If it is not treated, cardiovascular disease can bring on a fatal heart attack.

Hypertensive heart disease is caused by chronic, elevated blood pressure. When the blood pressure rises, the heart must work harder to move blood through the circulatory system. Chronic hypertension thickens and stiffens the heart muscles. This causes a wide range of physical symptoms and raises the chances of a stroke, kidney disease, or heart failure. According to the 2007 report by the Centers for Disease Control and Prevention, of 2.4 million deaths in the United States in 2004, high blood pressure was the contributing cause of death in 300,000 cases.

The pumping of blood through the heart can be temporarily stopped or interrupted. This brings cardiac arrythmia, a change in the normal rhythm of the heart. Most people occasionally feel their heart skip a beat, or suddenly beat more strongly than usual. In most cases, there is nothing dangerous or unusual about a sudden palpitation. Others suffering from arrhythmia have a chronically weak or irregular heartbeat that affects the movement of blood through the body. This can bring about heart disease or a heart attack.

Risk Factors

Researchers have identified several uncontrollable risk factors for heart disease. Age is one of the most important. After age 65, the risk of heart disease increases for men and women and throughout the population. Men are at greater risk than women, at any age. Heredity also plays a part; people with a history of heart attacks in their family are more likely to suffer from heart disease. African Americans are more susceptible to hypertension—one of the most important causes of heart trouble—than Caucasians.

Controllable risk factors include obesity and drinking too much alcohol. For tobacco smokers, the risk of heart attack is two to four times higher. A rise in blood cholesterol level, caused by heredity, diet, or disease, is another important risk factor, as is physical inactivity. Also, taking prescribed medications is essential to controlling disease.

HEART STRESSORS

Different kinds of stress affect the heart. Physical stress, for one, results from exercise, when the heart rate increases and remains elevated for some time. This is a good form of stress, one that improves the function of the heart and the circulatory system. A *lack* of physical stress on the heart—a completely sedentary lifestyle—actually increases the risk of heart disease. However, doctors advise people suffering from heart disease to avoid heavy physical stress. In people with coronary artery disease, too much stress on the heart and the arteries supplying blood to the body can make a heart attack more likely.

Fact Or Fiction?

Teenagers don't get heart attacks.

The Facts: Unless they are suffering from a hereditary heart condition, teenagers are largely free of the factors that contribute to heart attacks—including a buildup of high cholesterol, hypertension, diabetes, and obesity. Their arteries are still in good condition and have not yet had the plaque buildup that contributes to blockage and heart disease. As they get older, however, and begin unhealthy behaviors such as smoking, poor diet, and lack of exercise, their risk for heart attack increases.

Emotional Stress and the Heart

Sudden emergency situations such as an earthquake or fire can flood a body with stress hormones to such a level that a sudden heart attack is more likely. It is common knowledge among paramedics and emergency workers that people in a life-or-death situation can suffer a damaging, or fatal, heart attack.

People with sudden, difficult life changes such as the death of a family member are also more vulnerable to heart disease and heart attacks. Those who suffer intense emotional distress as a result of their work or home situations, and who suffer anger, **anxiety,** or depression, also tend to experience more heart trouble.

The body undergoes a direct physical reaction to a bout of emotional stress by releasing stress hormones such as adrenaline into the bloodstream. Adrenaline causes the blood to clot more easily—an adaptation that allows humans in emergency situations to recover more quickly from wounds. However, blood that clots more easily also places more stress on the heart.

Another important stress reaction caused by adrenaline is the constriction of blood vessels. This reaction limits the amount of blood moving to the extremities, which is why when stressed, hands and feet can feel cold. Constricted blood vessels also stress the circulatory system and the heart. When chronic emotional stress is present, the heart is exposed to stressors and symptoms that impede its ability to function normally.

Of course, not all emotional stress is bad. A certain level of stress in a job situation, for example, is stimulating to most people, while other people seem even to thrive on stress. For some, a vacation or holiday that promises a lack of stress and pressure can be depressing. For others, a break from stress is absolutely necessary, for both physical and mental well-being.

The difference is control. Those who feel in control of their situation tend to welcome a certain amount of stress. Those who have little or no control over their work or school lives, their home situation or their family life, seek to avoid stress as much as possible and suffer more from it when it occurs.

Fact Or Fiction?

Aspirin can stop a heart attack.

The Facts: Aspirin has the effect of decreasing the "stickiness" of blood platelets, which are small cells that clot the blood and can contribute to a heart attack. Chewed aspirin works the fastest—in just a matter of minutes. To prevent a heart attack in the future, doctors recommend taking a single aspirin a day.

The Coronary-Prone Type A

In the early 1960s, researchers began to take a closer look at the link between emotional states and heart disease. The researchers Mike Friedman and Ray Rosenman challenged the conventional medical wisdom that heart disease was caused by blockage of the arteries as a result of poor diet and a rise in blood cholesterol. They believed there could be social and cultural factors at work. They studied the incidence of heart disease in different regions of the world, including the United States, Mexico, and northern and southern Italy. They published their findings in the *Journal of the American Medical Association.*

In their research, carried out over several years, Friedman and Rosenman noted that men and women had different rates of heart disease in different geographic regions. Most of the heart attacks in the United States occurred in men. In Mexico and in southern Italy, men and women had equal rates. In northern Italy, men had four times the rate of heart disease as women.

Because there was no difference in environment or diet between males and females living in the same region, something else had to be at work. The researchers' concluded that gender roles, social expectations, and attitudes toward work made the difference. The concept of type A and type B personalities emerged.

Type A personalities were those considered driven and confrontational at work, more prone to anger and hostility, and susceptible to a stress reaction. Type A persons place higher expectations on themselves and seek to achieve constantly greater production from their work. They may feel a sense of guilt during off-hours or while on vacation. They are more competitive and have a greater need for recognition.

It is widely recognized that type A people suffer more heart problems than Type B people, who approach work expecting less from themselves and from others. One's attitude and interaction with others plays a key role. Type A personalities bring their work attitude to life in general and to all of their personal encounters. They are more impatient in conversation and experience more frequent episodes of anger, confrontation, physical stress, and hypertension. Even a minor episode of stress brings a surge of adrenaline and an unhealthy change in the body's blood chemistry.

Type B personalities better handle stress, although they are also more sensitive to it. They tend to defuse a confrontation and seek an immediate reduction in the stress level. They are not as driven to achievement, or high productivity, and do not place as high demands on themselves and on others. They also tend to be less physically active and may exhibit outer signs of inner stress: facial or speech tics, fidgeting, and so on.

STRESS, BEHAVIOR, AND THE HEART

Stress can bring about behavior that is bad for the heart. A person under a lot of stress may not pay much attention to overall health. A heavy load of work at school or at a job, for example, can stop a person from regular exercise. Stress can cause people to overeat, get less sleep, and turn to smoking and alcohol for relief. All of these actions raise either blood pressure or cholesterol, increasing the risk of a heart attack or heart disease.

There are also social factors that go into the risk of heart disease. People who are isolated from others and have a limited support network have a higher chance of having a heart attack. Those who have fewer dependents and on whom fewer family members or friends depend likewise have more heart trouble. The cause may be a more limited ability to share stress with others and thus defuse its mental and physical effects.

Q & A

Question: What are the signs of a heart attack?

Answer: The following are signs of a heart attack, when the passage of blood through the heart is partially or completely blocked: chest pains or pressure in the center of the chest that lasts more than a few minutes, shortness of breath, pain in the upper body, nausea, cold sweats, and dizziness. Most attacks are sudden and intense, but some start slowly.

A Stressful Modern Pace

Even as medical technology improves, heart disease remains a serious health problem—especially in modern industrialized nations with a generally faster pace of life. The speed of change in high-tech nations and their high incidence of heart disease may be more than a coincidence. With machines and technology moving faster than ever before, people are better able to undertake more tasks and, as a result, also are expected to finish them sooner. Research has shown a direct and immediate effect of mental stress on the heart's ability to move blood. In one test carried out at the University of Florida and described in the *Journal of the American College of Cardiology,* a group of cardiac patients were asked to imagine a stressful situation. They were then asked to give a short speech explaining how they would deal with the situation. Researchers injected a tracer into their bloodstream that measured blood flow through the heart. Six out of 29 experienced a bout of ischemia, decreased blood flow through the heart muscle, even though they felt no other symptoms of heart attack, such as chest pain or arrhythmia.

The study confirms what researchers have been suspecting since the concept of types A and B arose: There is a strong connection between mind and body when it comes to experiencing stress and to managing our reactions.

See also: Blood Pressure and Stress; Exercise and Stress; Gender and Stress; Treatment; Workplace Stress

FURTHER READING

Phibbs, Brendan. *The Human Heart: A Basic Guide to Heart Disease.* Philadelphia: Lippincott, Williams & Wilkins, 2007.

Wulsin, Lawson R. *Treating the Aching Heart: A Guide to Depression, Stress, and Heart Disease.* Nashville, Tenn.: Vanderbilt University Press, 2007.

■ STRESS IN SCHOOL

Sources of physical and emotional conflict that are common experiences of students of all ages, beginning in about middle school and arising from academics, family pressures, and social interactions at or related to school. The expectations of parents, teachers, and friends combine to place a heavy burden on many students, who are also undergoing important physical changes. A student experiencing stress may not understand or be able to identify the source of physical and emotional stress symptoms nor know of any healthful therapies that may provide coping mechanisms.

ACADEMIC STRESS

Stress at school begins with academic pressure. In an all-day schedule of different classes, the mind's focus must constantly shift from one subject to the next. Each class introduces concepts and information new to the student, who has little time to assimilate that information. Teachers expect class participation and challenge students to provide answers or solve new problems on the spot. Surprise tests may be trouble for an unprepared student at any time. Classroom distractions, such as disciplinary action by the teacher and random chatter by other students, also make it difficult to focus.

Time for doing academic work within the school walls is limited, and most students have study hall or free time of only an hour. Work brought home lengthens the school day, and each class may require a different home assignment. In this way, the mental stress associated with learning, reading, writing, and problem solving continues without relief for most of a student's waking hours.

Few students practice any kind of time budgeting or planning. Without a schedule of when and how to prepare homework, the academic workload becomes a heavy burden, causing more worry and anxiety over available time. Pressure from parents to finish work, as well as to pursue other interests such as music, art, or athletics, increases the mental and physical burden.

When children begin their school careers, most have lived free of what adults know as stress. In elementary school, children become accustomed to a day divided into blocks of time, devoted to classroom work, recess, gym class, or lunch. Although they soon begin doing homework and taking tests, by the time they enter middle school, students still experience relatively little awareness of mental and physical stress. They know little about the symptoms of stress, unless they see these symptoms in parents or teachers. Unless children have received advice from parents or counseling from a doctor or therapist, they know little or nothing about useful stress management techniques.

As they grow older, students are subject to the higher expectations of authority figures and anxiety over exams, homework deadlines, and the opinions of their peers. While most tend to seek out the approval of and strive to earn the high grades rewarded by teachers, students also experience the desire to fit in and be accepted by peers. These two goals are often mutually exclusive. A high achiever may feel like an outcast among friends who pay little attention to grades or who feel that striving for high grades is uncool. Also, as high school students near college age, they experience more pressure to perform academically—in classes and on college entrance examinations. Unless school counselors, health class teachers, or parents talk specifically with teenage students about stress, the normal coping mechanisms for those who suffer from high levels of stress remain out of reach.

Stress in College

Negative reactions to stressful events often worsen in college. Students entering college are often leaving behind their friends and family, moving to a location away from home, and gradually losing touch with most of the people they once knew. For the first time they are living on their own, facing a heavier workload and more difficult academics, with no parents or old friends to assist them.

College also places the stress of choice on students. Faced with a multitude of available classes, they must decide what and how they want to study. They must select a major and eventually prepare for graduate school or for work. These crucial decisions are difficult to make.

College students may cope with stress in unhealthy ways—drinking and partying without sleep; overeating, or eating unhealthy food; doing minimal physical exercise. These activities worsen physical health and mental focus.

Such problems drive some students to eventually drop out of college and seek a more manageable environment in the form of a job with structure, straightforward duties, and close supervision by managers. Although 60 percent of high school seniors continue to college, about half of all college students drop out before completing their degree.

SOCIAL AND FAMILY STRESSORS

At the same time that students feel the pressure of academic demands, peer pressure is at work as well. Students in high school function in a charged atmosphere, completely foreign to their earlier school experience. The school places together a large group of young strangers through most of the day, a situation that requires the ability to make and keep acquaintances with others, deal with rivalries and jealousies, dress and behave according to popular fashion, and maintain one's self-respect. Friendships are made and broken; cliques form to exclude outsiders; individuals emerge as leaders or followers. The intense self-attention of a young child must begin to turn outward, without much guidance or support from anyone. These situations can result in feelings of isolation and helplessness.

Parents and siblings are also sources of stress. Parents have high expectations of their children and often measure their own success in life through the academic achievements of their children. This can bring pressure at home to achieve high grades, take on a heavy schedule of classes, take part in extracurricular activities, and compete for academic honors. The desire of children to please parents can result in further stress and anxiety to a student who is already coping with social and academic pressures at school.

A research study done in Los Angeles and published in the journal *Child Development* found that stress at home can affect school life and vice versa. The study examined 589 ninth graders from three schools, who kept diaries for two weeks, checking off lists of various stressful issues they may have experienced each day. When difficulties occurred at home, researchers found, there were problems immediately at school, either with attendance or classroom work. Stress at school also spilled over into the home situation. A separate study found that ninth graders who began high school with a high level of stress went through the next year with academic problems, up to and including their senior years.

TEENS SPEAK

Issues at Home

There's a lot of fighting going on at home. My parents argue constantly about everything you can think of: money, cars, work, and especially the house. They don't see eye to eye on anything, and I sometimes wonder why they got married in the first place.

When I get to school I keep thinking about it. I remember everything that everyone said. Then I try to figure out whether I could have said something to stop all the fighting. It's hard to concentrate in class, and I feel myself getting nervous and stressed. On the days after a bad night, I'm not in the mood to study at all. When I get home there's not much peace and quiet, so I can't get my homework done.

I told my teacher about it. She said she understood and would have my parents come in for a meeting. I said, better wait. I told her I wasn't sure that was a good idea. If she does that, then I'll be the one that caused another problem—

having to come in to see the teacher, as if my parents were in some kind of trouble with the school. But if things keep going the way they are, that's just what I'm going to do.

COPING WITH SCHOOL STRESS

Stress at school manifests itself in different ways for each individual. An inability to concentrate, either at school or at home, is a sign of growing mental stress, which also can cause sleeplessness, a lack of appetite, and lack of interest in friends and family. Students facing a deadline for an assignment may experience fatigue and drowsiness, as well as an inability to concentrate. For some, the day of a final exam may bring intense anxiety and even physical illness.

There are many simple, practical ways of coping with stress. The most effective are work habits that a student can learn with little effort. These include straightforward life management skills such as eating well, allowing enough time for sleep, and regular exercise.

Work and Time Budgeting

To lighten the burden of work, students should budget their time using a daily planner. Many schools provide or require one. The planner allows the student to see exactly what work is required, day by day, and to set appointments to meet deadlines and prepare for upcoming exams.

If difficult schoolwork itself is causing intense stress, students need tutoring from teachers. A problem difficult to solve becomes easier if someone who knows the subject well can explain it. Although this can be difficult in a classroom, teachers should be available at some time during the day or immediately after school to meet with the student one-on-one and review the work. Also, if an assignment is taking too long to complete or an emergency comes up, a teacher will often grant a short extension, as long as missing deadlines does not become a habit. If a student is taking a class that is simply too advanced, schools will sometimes allow that student to transfer to an easier one.

Organization

Organization of work is another very effective means of coping with academic stress. This requires keeping books and folders separate and labeled for each class. Students also should pay attention to their important supplies, calculators, pencils, and notebooks. Losing material is the most common **stressor** affecting students, and it usually arises from poor organization.

Homework should also be prioritized. The most important work is usually that due the soonest. Students should be clear on due dates, as noted in their planners. Tackling assignments one at a time and in order of importance will divide the work into manageable tasks and ease the heavy burden. For even more careful organization, students can estimate how much time each assignment will take and plan their time accordingly. Long-term assignments such as term papers can be broken down into separate tasks: research, drafting, revising.

Fact Or Fiction?

Stress causes acne.

The Facts: The release of *stress hormones* by the adrenal glands during the "fight-or-flight" response causes a chemical chain reaction in the body. Eventually the overproduction of hormones affects the sebaceous glands, which lie at the base of hair follicles. These glands release an oily substance known as sebum, which travels up the hair follicles, clogs the pores of the skin, and can begin an acne breakout.

Keeping Perspective

The psychological burden of high academic and social stress at school can be lessened by improving mental attitude. It helps to keep perspective on the work and understand that everyone around you is facing a similar situation. Students should also avoid negative buzz-words—*never, impossible, hard,*—that will place mental blocks in the way of success. Positive affirmations made silently can help: "I can do this work." "This assignment will be done by tomorrow." "This class is not so difficult." Visualizations are also useful. The student simply imagines completing the work and turning it in on time or giving a presentation to an appreciative class (and teacher).

Fact Or Fiction?

Smoking pot relieves your stress level.

The Facts: Smoking marijuana will cause much more stress, both physical and mental, than it solves. Pot smoking is hard on the lungs, heart, and circulatory system. It affects short-term memory, attention span, and the ability to work through a problem in logic or math. The failing grade on a paper or test that results will undoubtedly raise stress levels, as will eventual feelings of paranoia and lack of self-confidence that often occur after long-term, *chronic* marijuana use.

A sense of optimism can be hard to develop. Worries over assignments and social life can easily bring on a negative state of mind, in which one imagines only a bad outcome. To reverse the negative thinking, a student can start by imagining a long-term future, one in which his or her goals are finally achieved. Learning to replace negative thoughts with positive messages and images will help bring about this better outcome.

The Working Environment
A better focus on the work at hand is also helpful. Students must control distractions such as television, text messaging, and the Internet. The best way to limit the time devoted to them is to delay a distraction until the work is finished.

The working environment is also crucial to reducing stress. The room should be quiet, and all interruptions banished. If possible, meeting with another student with the same assignment and working together sometimes can get the task finished in a much shorter time. This allows each person to solve a single, manageable part of the assignment and reduces the amount of work that the other would have to get done on his or her own.

Taking a break in the middle of a homework session also will help reduce the stress caused by worry and constant concentration. A walk around the block may clear the head and allow the mind, either consciously or subconsciously, to focus on the problem at hand. If a problem seems unsolvable, or writer's block arises, a full night's sleep (during which the mind continues to process information) will often supply the answer in the morning.

Simple Stress Management Methods
There are routines and methods for coping directly with stress. The practice of yoga is one, in which students assume a series of postures and simultaneously clear their minds of distracting thoughts and images. The yoga session usually ends with an enhanced sense of calm and readiness to face challenges.

Meditation is another effective stress management technique. In a quiet room, a person meditating concentrates on a single sound or syllable, repeated silently under steady, controlled breathing. The goal is to reach a state of mind in which no exterior thoughts or worries intrude. Although meditation, like yoga, takes practice, it can help reduce stress and even relieve the physical symptoms that may accompany stress.

See also: Performance Anxiety; Stress and the Environment; Stress and the Family; Types of Stress

FURTHER READING

Belknap, Martha. *Stress Relief for Kids: Taming Your Dragons.* Duluth, Minn.: Whole Person Associates, 2006.

Bugni, Patrick. *The Stress Kitchen: Why Kids Hate School and What We Can Do to Change It.* Bloomington, Ind.: Author House, 2005.

White, Dr. Tania. *Stress Management for Schools.* Lulu.com, 2008.

■ STRESS MANAGEMENT TECHNIQUES

Methods of controlling our mental and physical reactions to particular events. These range from ancient traditional practices such as prayer and meditation to an integrated modern approach that includes physical exercises, mental training, diet, and medications. Because stress is an unavoidable part of our lives, stress management has become a health industry. Self-help books and Web sites suggesting effective stress management methods are readily available, as are therapists and counselors who specialize in this relatively new field of study.

Stress management techniques can be divided into two broad categories: physical and mental. Some methods can be integrated easily into daily life: basic healthy habits of sleep, diet, regular exercise, and work or school routines that counteract the events that arise from living and working day to day. Other techniques must be practiced and in many cases coached; some are the object of lifelong study.

PHYSICAL STRESS MANAGEMENT

There are several benefits of physical stress management techniques or those associated with movement, exercise, and physical training.

Repetitive and controlled movement of the body helps many people attain a state of calm and concentration and banish the sources of stress found in work, school, or the home. The health benefits of regular exercise include improvements in alertness, lowered blood pressure, weight loss, better circulation, and improved sleep—all helpful in combating the physical effects of stress. Mental stress management techniques such as meditation often make up an important element of these methods.

Exercise

A regular exercise routine is one of the most effective ways to manage stress. Jogging, walking, bicycling, and swimming are all excellent ways to lessen physical tension and reduce anxiety and depression. People can exercise without competing, alone or in combination with meditation or other stress-fighting mental techniques.

An exercise routine takes one directly out of a stressful environment and away from the situations that may be causing stress, whether at home or at school. Exercise also improves overall fitness and physical health by improving lung capacity, working and strengthening the heart and blood vessels, and toning up the muscles. Good health allows one to deal better with challenging events as they arise and recover one's emotional balance quickly.

Qigong and Tai Chi

Qigong is a Chinese method of combining simple physical movement and breathing techniques with meditation. The goal is to help cure illness, combat stress, and enhance the circulation of essential *qi,* or life force, within the body. Within China, *qigong* is recognized as an important medical discipline and is the subject of studies and research papers. *Qigong* has also attracted the attention of stress management professionals in the western world.

Qigong is practiced in thousands of different ways by people in all walks of life. There are religious, medical, and martial-arts forms. *Qigong* movements can be performed indoors or outside, while standing or sitting. In some forms of *qigong,* the body goes through a series of strictly controlled movements while the practitioner concentrates on words or concepts that help him or her keep a mental focus. In one popular form known as *baduanjin,* the body goes through eight very specific postures, which are intended to direct *qi* through the body's eight different channels or "meridians."

Tai chi is another form of Chinese exercise, consisting of controlled movements that are done slowly enough to develop balance, coordination, strength, and deep concentration. There are five major schools of tai chi movements, each broken down in several different approaches that combine the postures and forms in different ways and for different purposes.

Yoga

In a yoga class, a teacher instructs a group of people in a series of postures, some easy and some more challenging, which are designed to develop balance, strength, and flexibility. Each posture is given a name, and as students move from one to the next each student strives to achieve a sense of balance and flow.

Yoga classes have become a popular way for people to cope with stress as the deep concentration required by yoga postures has the effect of crowding out external sources of anxiety. Advocates of yoga as a stress management tool claim that it has a direct effect on muscle tone and flexibility, easing the muscles and joints into a relaxed state.

There are different schools of yoga, some easy and some very difficult. It takes no previous training to join a yoga class, however, as everyone is encouraged to proceed at his or her own pace and ability level.

Guided Physical Relaxation

Another simple method of coping with stress is the practice of guided physical relaxation. Progressive Muscle Relaxation (PMR), which was first developed in the 1930s, is one of the simplest relaxation techniques and can be practiced at home. In a daily PMR session, the individual sits in a comfortable position in a quiet room. He or she goes through the parts of the body, from the feet to the head, tensing and then relaxing the muscles in each part. The most common sequence begins at the feet and progresses as follows:

Right foot

Right lower leg and foot

Entire right leg

Left foot

Left lower leg and foot

Entire left leg

Right hand

Right forearm and hand

Entire right arm

Left hand

Left forearm and hand

Entire left arm

Abdomen

Chest

Neck and shoulders

Face

The practice of PMR trains the body to relax muscles that have been tensed, either by work or by a stressful social situation. By doing PMR every day, a person gradually develops the ability to reduce the physical reaction to a source of stress.

A similar method of physical relaxation is "autogenic" training, a method of creating sensations in the body. This technique was developed by the German psychologist Johannes Schultz in the early 1930s. Autogenic training is a form of autosuggestion, in which an individual controls breathing while repeating silently a physical sensation to be induced: "My right arm is getting heavy," for example, followed by "my left arm is getting heavy." The autogenic session ends with a simple conclusion such as, "I feel supremely calm." The technique demands a period of training in its use as the combinations grow more complex and the sessions get longer. Autogenic training has been shown to result in greater control over the body, reduced stress, and even the conquest of harmful addictions such as alcoholism.

Biofeedback gained popularity during the 1970s as another method of stress control. In a biofeedback lab, monitoring equipment is set up to gauge the body's physical reactions to stress, which include raised heart rate and blood pressure, brain activity, and muscle tension. With training, these can be controlled. To do so, the individual can use techniques of breathing, guided meditations, Progressive Muscle Relaxation, or any other technique that seems effective. The goal is to help the individual gain some control over the **autonomic nervous system,** which automatically reacts to stress. Biofeedback sessions are usually held under the supervision of a physician or psychologist trained in the use of the monitoring equipment.

MENTAL STRESS MANAGEMENT

Mental stress management techniques are exercises carried out by conscious thought and imagination. Some are simple enough to learn alone and use at home or anywhere one finds a quiet place with no distractions. Others are more complex and require some form of training, as well as the guidance of an instructor or counselor. The ultimate goal of these techniques is control of the mental and physical reactions to events and to ease the anxiety that arises when anticipating stressful situations.

Meditation

Meditation has long been one of the most popular methods of concentration and relaxation. In many religions, contemplation and mental focus are encouraged as ways of attaining peace of mind and, as a result, spiritual insight. Meditation can be carried out in a great variety of ways. There are few rules associated with a meditation session, nor is there a particular setting or any sort of equipment required. One needs only a room or space free of distractions. Every person practicing a form of meditation will develop his or her own methods and habits.

The meditation session begins with a controlled relaxation of the body and a series of deep breaths that help to calm and focus the mind. A simple sound or syllable is repeated, silently or out loud, until the mind has reached total concentration on that sound. The idea of meditation is to banish all exterior stimuli and control the jumble of thoughts, worries, and memories that crowd the conscious mind.

The Relaxation Response

The relaxation response is a variation on the idea of meditation, developed by Dr. Herbert Benson, a professor of medicine at Harvard. The goal of the relaxation response is to create a body state in which the muscles and circulatory system attain a state of complete relaxation and the autonomic system in charge of the "fight-or-flight" response is temporarily shut down.

The relaxation response begins by closing the eyes, then relaxing the parts of the body from the feet to the head, one by one. The breath is steady and controlled, with the word *one* repeated after each exhale. This controlled breathing continues for 10 minutes; if a distracting thought or image arrives, it is banished with the next repetition of *one*. The body is then allowed to gradually return to its normal settings.

Guided Imagery

In guided imagery, the individual brings a series of calming images to mind, while relaxing the body in a comfortable position and controlling breathing. The images can be of anything the individual finds pleasant and can include sensations of sound, scent, and texture.

Guided imagery scripts often include a series of directions or questions. By carefully examining the physical and mental reactions to stress, the script seeks to resolve anger, for example, or banish the fear of a future stress-inducing challenge such as speaking in public. The script may end with a series of affirmations, positive statements made to confirm that one is in control of one's emotions and that the session has been successful. For example:

1. I acknowledge that I am feeling angry right now and accept the way I feel.
2. I have the power to control my reactions.
3. I can fully experience this anger, yet wait before I take action.
4. I can feel angry but calm and in control at the same time.
5. It's okay to feel angry.

LIFE MANAGEMENT

People dealing with stress can take some simple steps to rid themselves of bad habits, both physical and mental, and improve their overall health and state of mind. The most basic of these life skills is time management. Although everyone must undertake certain tasks, these can be prioritized and carefully scheduled so that everyday obligations do not turn into an unmanageable overload. Using a planner, people can avoid time conflicts when agreeing to tasks and cancel or postpone those for which they cannot set aside any time. By reserving time each day for necessary tasks such as answering phone messages or e-mail, the problem of procrastination can also be solved.

Organization

Stress also can be managed with the organization and control of one's physical environment. Clutter on a desk or work space leads to misplaced papers or tools, a very common source of stress. As a scheduled task, organizing a work space can be done on a regular basis, for example at the end of the day. An exterior source of stress, such as the television news, may also be eliminated or changed so that its negative qualities are reduced. Giving more time to a longer but calmer traffic route, for example, is one way of overcoming commuter stress. Shopping or doing chores in the weekday mornings, rather than on weekends, calms the stress of mall crowds, post office lines, and parking lot snarls.

Support networks

The use of a support network of friends and family can also go a long way toward alleviating sources of stress. Many studies have pointed to the benefits of a social network, finding that a group of friends can improve the management of stress and even has long-term physical benefits such as reducing blood pressure and improving brain function. Friends allow one another to vent their frustrations and fears; psychologists and counselors depend on the fact that the verbalization of inner conflict goes a long way to relieving it. Similarly, people who tend to be sources of stress, for whatever reason, can be avoided or, if that is impossible, their presence channeled into a specific day or kept to a limited block of time.

Attitude

Personal attitude adjustment is another key weapon in managing stress, although it can be one of the most difficult. Negative thoughts and worries can have a physical effect, triggering the "fight-or-flight" mechanism and setting off the physical effects of stress hormones. For this reason, simple control of the conscious mind can be a major step toward reducing stress.

Finding perspective

A sense of obligation to a coach at school or a manager at work, for example, can develop into a need for perfectionism, but it can be resolved by meeting with the coach or the boss and setting goals that are easier to achieve. Personal and family problems can be reframed into a new perspective and turned into opportunities for achievement. Gaining a sense of perspective, therefore, also can alleviate stress. Those who suffer from pressured lives are often counseled to reflect on their achievements and to focus on a future date when a stressful situation will be resolved and forgotten.

Simple acceptance of a bad outcome can also help resolve stress. Situations such as the health problems of friends or family members, the loss suffered by a favorite sports team, or the effects of a weak economy lay outside of one's control. Instead of dwelling on these events and attempting to visualize a better outcome, the reality of the situation can be faced, fully understood, and finally accepted. Anger can be replaced with resignation and the anticipation of positive events in the future. Dwelling on the past and regretting events that cannot be changed can be a continual source of harmful emotional stress that can be resolved with adjusted attitudes and finding a sense of perspective.

See also: Exercise and Stress; Meditation; Relaxation Therapies; Treatment

FURTHER READING

Charlesworth, Edward A., and Ronald G. Nathan. *Stress Management: A Comprehensive Guide to Wellness.* New York: Ballantine Books, 2004.

Davis, Martha. *The Relaxation and Stress Reduction Workbook.* Oakland, Calif.: New Harbinger Publications, 2008.

Lehrer, Paul M. *Principles and Practice of Stress Management.* Third Edition. New York: The Guilford Press, 2008.

■ STRESS RATING SCALES

Methods of rating the impact of varying types of stress, or of the degree of chronic stress present. Stress rating scales are used by physicians and psychologists to measure the amount of stress their patients are experiencing and how certain events may be affecting their patients' physical and mental health. Although there are dozens of stress rating systems, the Social Readjustment Rating Scale developed by Thomas Holmes and Richard Rahe in the 1960s remains the most widely used stress rating method.

HOLMES-RAHE SCALE

Stress has been the subject of research and measurement since the term *stress* was coined in 1936 by Hans Selye, a professor at McGill University in Montreal; Selye referred to stress at that time as a "nonspecific response of the body to a demand." As stress became a popular field of medical research in the 1960s, the first "stress scale" was developed to aid in that research by two psychiatrists, Thomas Holmes and Richard Rahe. They rated a series of 43 stressful life events on a scale of 1 to 100. The higher the number, the more stressful the event, and, Holmes and Rahe suspected, the more severe the potential impact of the stress on physical health. They called their device the Social Readjustment Rating Scale, or SRSS.

On the Holmes-Rahe scale, the death of a spouse rates as the most stressful event possible, with a rating of 100. Divorce rates 73, and marital separation 65. Further down the scale of stressors are pregnancy (40), a child's leaving the home (29), boss trouble (23), and changing schools (20). The mildest events are Christmas holiday stress (12), and a "minor violation of the law," at 11.

To test the validity of their scale, Holmes and Rahe ran several research experiments by administering it to various groups in various locales. One such survey administered the SRSS to 5,000 patients. The subjects checked the events that had occurred in their own lives and added up the rating numbers Holmes and Rahe had associated with these events. The study found that there was a positive correlation of higher stress ratings to physical illness.

Another study was carried out in 1970 on a group of 2,500 members of the U.S. Navy. A similar correlation was found in the Holmes-Rahe overall stress rating as a predictor of future illness (determined in this case by visits to a navy doctor or medical unit). The Holmes-Rahe stress scale also was tested on people of different nations all over the world, and it was found to have a universal, cross-cultural application to the effect of stress on the human body.

The Holmes-Rahe scale is still in use by psychiatrists and therapists. Patients review the list, marking every event they have experienced over the past 12 months. The health-care professional then adds up the numbers that correlate to each event. A score of 150 or less indicates a level of positive stress and low risk to physical health. A score between 150 and 300 indicates a more serious impact of stress and an even higher chance of illness. A score of more than 300 indicates a high risk of physical effects and/or illnesses as the result of stressful events.

USING THE HOLMES-RAHE SCALE

There are wide variations of reactions to stress, and different people use different coping mechanisms. In some, a high stress score might inevitably lead to ill health, while others might have a higher tolerance to the combination of stressors in their lives. Some personalities, in fact, thrive on moderate levels of stress. Some individuals tolerate criticism and trouble with the boss, for example, without experiencing stress in either a psychological or physical sense. Others feel a high degree of stress when confronted by relatively minor changes or challenges such as confrontation with a boss or a spouse or even a stranger. Diet, exercise, social interactions, and other exterior factors, as well as one's age and overall state of health, also play a role in the body's response to stress.

While low stress ratings may be desirable for overall health, a zero stress rating, in modern industrialized society, is probably impossible to achieve as long as one has interactions with family, friends, and work colleagues. Some researchers have also pointed out that a minimal level of stress, or the good stress known as eustress, is desirable. A certain amount of "positive stress," as might be indicated by a Holmes-Rahe scale measure of 150 or below, means that an individual is appropriately confronting certain life challenges, which are often rewarding and usually necessary for personal development.

High stress scores would show a need to take some positive action to change one's life, work, and/or circumstances. For a patient with a high score, a physician would recommend a complete review of lifestyle, family, and work situations. He or she would advise that changes be made where possible to reduce the stressors already present.

To lessen the risks of moderate stress, a patient would be advised to avoid or postpone, if possible, certain events that are raising the stress score. Of course some events are out of one's control and cannot be avoided. Others such as taking out a mortgage (stress rating 32) or a change in recreation (19) at least can be postponed. As positive action, the doctor might also suggest one or several stress management techniques such as meditation, regular yoga classes, physical exercise, and a change in diet and sleep habits.

MORE RECENT STRESS SCALES

Since the creation of the Holmes-Rahe scale, many variations have been developed. Some are measures of stress in the general population, while others are geared to specific occupations, such as the Index of Teaching Stress, the Nurse Stress Index, and the Occupational Stress

DID YOU KNOW?

Taking the Holmes-Rahe Stress Scale

Life Event—Adults	Life Change Units
Death of a spouse	100
Divorce	73
Marital separation	65
Imprisonment	63
Death of a close family member	63
Personal injury or illness	53
Marriage	50
Dismissal from work	47
Marital reconciliation	45
Retirement	45
Change in health of family member	44
Pregnancy	40
Sexual difficulties	39
Gain a new family member	39
Business readjustment	39
Change in financial state	38
Change in frequency of arguments	35
Major mortgage	32
Foreclosure of mortgage or loan	30
Change in responsibilities at work	29
Child leaving home	29
Trouble with in-laws	29
Outstanding personal achievement	28
Spouse starts or stops work	26
Begin or end school	26
Change in living conditions	25
Revision of personal habits	24
Trouble with boss	23
Change in working hours or conditions	20
Change in residence	20
Change in schools	20
Change in recreation	19
Change in church activities	19

Holmes–Rahe Stress Scale *(continued)*

Change in social activities	18
Minor mortgage or loan	17
Change in sleeping habits	16
Change in number of family reunions	15
Change in eating habits	15
Vacation	13
Christmas	12
Minor violation of law	11

Life Event—Adolescents	Life Change Units
Getting married	101
Unwed pregnancy	92
Death of parent	87
Acquiring a visible deformity	81
Divorce of parents	77
Fathering an unwed pregnancy	77
Becoming involved with drugs or alcohol	76
Jail sentence of parent for over one year	75
Marital separation of parents	69
Death of a brother or sister	68
Change in acceptance by peers	67
Pregnancy of unwed sister	64
Discovery of being an adopted child	63
Marriage of parent to stepparent	63
Death of a close friend	63
Having a visible congenital deformity	62
Serious illness requiring hospitalization	58
Failure of a grade in school	56
Not making an extracurricular activity	55
Hospitalization of a parent	55
Jail sentence of parent for more than 30 days	53
Breaking up with boyfriend or girlfriend	53
Beginning to date	51
Suspension from school	50

(continues)

Holmes–Rahe Stress Scale *(continued)*

Birth of a brother or sister	50
Increase in arguments between parents	47
Loss of job by parent	46
Outstanding personal achievement	46
Change in parent's financial status	45
Accepted at college of choice	43
Being a senior in high school	42
Hospitalization of a sibling	41
Increased absence of parent from home	38
Brother or sister leaving home	37
Addition of third adult to family	34
Becoming a full-fledged member of a church	31
Decrease in arguments between parents	27
Decrease in arguments with parents	26
Mother or father beginning work	26

If you are 18 or under, in the scale for adolescents, mark each life event that has occurred within the past 12 months. Add up the numbers corresponding to the events marked. A score of 300 or above indicates a high concentration of stressors, which pose a relatively high risk to physical and psychological health. A score between 150 and 300 indicates a moderate health risk, and a score of 150 or below indicates little health risk. Below 50 indicates an inadequate amount of "good stress," which brings motivation for personal growth and development.

Inventory. The occupational scales are widely used as a measure of the psychological health (and productivity) of a workforce in a particular location or company. Others are used by doctors or therapists trying to understand the root cause of an individual's physical or emotional symptoms. A few of these stress rating scales are described below.

Daily Stress Inventory
Another method of reporting stress is through the Daily Stress Inventory, a record of minor stressors experienced by people in their daily lives. The DSI lists 58 stressful events in the categories of interpersonal problems, personal competency, cognitive stressors, environmental hassles, and "varied stressors." Each event is rated on a scale of 1 ("occurred but was not stressful") to 7 ("made me panic"). The DSI can be applied in many different settings, from measuring satisfaction

in the workplace to medical research into the direct physical effects of stress.

Maslach Burnout Inventory

Developed by Christina Maslach, this inventory is a tool that attempts to assess the risk of job burnout: the feeling of exhaustion, fatigue, boredom, and frustration that can affect morale, lower productivity, and even lead to confrontations and violence in the workplace. The Maslach Burnout Inventory has not been well researched as to its accuracy or predictive power. However, it has been widely used in an informal way by company managements. The test attempts to predict emotional exhaustion; "depersonalization" (in which employees grow apathetic toward colleagues, clients, and customers); and sense of personal accomplishment and basic competence, an important measure of morale. The presence of burnout can mean lower productivity, higher absenteeism, a higher incidence of workplace accidents, and a higher rate of employee turnover—all costly events for company success.

Parenting Stress Index

Like many other stress scales, the Parenting Stress Index is a self-reporting tool that people can administer to themselves to gauge the amount of stress in their relationship with children from three months to 10 years old. The PSU has 101 items, which include various events and problems that occur between parents and children. The PSI has been extensively researched and shown to predict the future social adjustment of children. An extension of the PSI was later developed as the Stress Index for Parenting Adolescents.

Student Stress Rating Scale

As a Parents Stress Index came into existence, a Student Stress Rating Scale was also developed from the original Holmes-Rahe scale. The SSRS contained events that younger people are likely to experience, including "Divorce Between Parents," "Failing a Course," and "New Girlfriend or Boyfriend." The events are assigned a number between 1 and 100. As with the Holmes-Rahe scale, the numbers are added together and are correlated to risk of serious illness. In the Social Readjustment Rating Scale, published in the *Journal of Psychosomatic Research* in 1967, the developers of the scale cited the many different life events and situations that can bring about a stress overload on students as follows:

Difficult classes, poor time management, work overload, poor study skills, commuting to school, examinations and revision, difficulties with family members, dissatisfaction with course, poor relationship with tutors, significant people's expectations, fear of failure, financial difficulties, feelings of inadequacy, fear of unknown assessments, unsatisfactory accommodation, friends, roommates, poor communication skills, body image, diet and nutrition, lack of exercise, serious illness, [and/or a] death or tragedy in family.

The Perceived Stress Scale

A close relative of the Holmes-Rahe scale is the Perceived Stress Scale, or PSS. First published in the *Journal of Health and Social Behavior* in 1983, the scale measures stress in a slightly different way, by considering the individual's own appraisal of how severe the stress has been. By asking a series of 10 questions about how often the individual has felt a certain way in the last month, the PSS is intended to gauge to what degree people find their lives uncontrolled and unpredictable. The questions begin with: "In the last month, how often have you been upset because of something that happened unexpectedly?" The patient answers with a 0 if "Never" up to a 4 for "Very Often." Researchers have correlated high scores on the PSS to health problems and vulnerability to depression and anxiety.

SUBJECTIVE MEASURES

Since it was invented in the 1960s, the stress rating scale has become a popular tool in predicting and diagnosing the effects of psychological and physical stress. However, stress remains an imprecise and relatively subjective field of medical study. Responses given by a subject to a stress questionnaire do not represent an objective measure of stress in the same way that a thermometer, for example, gives a reading of body temperature or that an electronic monitor indicates heart rate. Instead, stress responses represent the subjects' own opinion or feelings about stressors present in their lives and the events they experience. Opinion can be affected by many outside factors and can vary over time. In correlating stress with physical symptoms, there is much more research to be done and, no doubt, to that end many more precise measuring tools will be developed in an effort to attain an objective measure of stress.

See also: Biology of Stress; Stress and the Environment; Stress and the Family; Stress at School; Types of Stress; Workplace Stress

FURTHER READING
Balamurugan, M., and D. Kumaran. "Development and Validation of Students' Stress Rating Scale (SSRS)." Available online. URL: http://www.eric.ed.gov/ERICWebPortal/custom/portlets/recordDetails/detailmini.jsp?_nfpb=true&_&ERICExtSearch_SearchValue_0=ED5 01881&ERICExtSearch _SearchType_0=no&accno=ED501881.
Cohen, Sheldon, Ronald C. Kessler, and Lynn Underwood Gordon, *Measuring Stress: A Guide for Health and Social Scientists.* New York: Oxford University Press, 1997.
Khan, Ada P., *Stress A-Z: A Sourcebook for Facing Everyday Challenges.* New York: Checkmark Books, 2000.
Zalaquett, Carlos P. and Richard J. Wood. *Evaluating Stress: A Book of Resources.* Lanham, Md.: Scarecrow Press, 1998.

■ TREATMENT

A course of action to fight illness or disorder that is specific to the symptoms of that illness. Severe stress has become a common illness. According to a 2007 Stress and Anxiety Disorders Survey, 48 percent of people who experience stress report that it affects their activities every day. The most common physical effects are a loss of sleep (68 percent); headaches (58 percent); upset stomach or nausea (49 percent); pounding heartbeat (40 percent); and back pain (35 percent).

When negative reactions to **stressors** become severe enough to affect one's physical health, professional treatment becomes a valuable option. Because everyone reacts differently to stress, doctors and counselors usually tailor each plan of treatment to the individual. These therapies can include stress management techniques, advice on lifestyle changes, and medication. The treatment will also vary with the age of a patient, the situation that is causing the stress, and whether the symptoms are psychological, physical, or a combination of both.

MEDICATION

Stress often results in mild physical symptoms for which people seek help from medical doctors. For tension headaches, doctors generally prescribe over-the-counter medications such as aspirin or ibuprofen. For digestive problems, patients may use antacids or laxatives. Certain herbs advertised as effective antistress medications are available in nutritional supplements. These include Saint-John's-wort, ginseng, valerian, lemon balm, and chamomile. These supplements are available over the counter without a prescription.

People suffering symptoms of stress often turn to alcohol or drugs in an attempt to "self-medicate" and relieve their symptoms. Doctors counseling someone who reports heavy stress will usually ask about alcohol or drug use, which can become habitual and create much more stress than these substances solve.

If stress develops into a case of panic attacks, **anxiety,** or **chronic depression,** doctors may prescribe medications such as Xanax or Valium. These drugs are designed to temporarily relieve psychological symptoms but are never prescribed for stress resulting from basic work or family pressures. These medications are not intended to "cure" since they provide relief from the symptoms of stress but cannot change the outside stressor.

Untreated physical symptoms, however, can become severe. Nervousness, shortness of breath, and a constant stress reaction can bring about heart problems and high blood pressure. If a patient has trouble sleeping at night or functioning during the day, a doctor may advise a more structured treatment plan, which includes rest, a break from work, or a course of therapy.

STRESS THERAPIES

Psychiatrists, who are medical doctors, are usually knowledgeable about treating stress and can prescribe appropriate medications combined with therapy. This is one form of treatment.

Another stress treatment is self-care. Counselors advise their patients to take positive actions to head off serious physical problems that will arise later if the stress is not resolved. This treatment consists of a combination of different approaches.

One important aspect of self-care is physical activity and regular exercise, which allow people to release pent-up energy, improve the body's physical condition, relax, and turn the mind away from the stressor. Counselors will also advise restful periods during the day and allowing enough time for sleep at night, a better diet, and taking a break from one's routine.

Stressed patients also can employ visualization and meditation as a course of treatment. Visualization is the use of peaceful imagery to turn the mind away from any situation causing a stress response. Meditation is a daily practice in which a person rests the body in a quiet room and focuses on a single sound or syllable to clear the mind of stressful thoughts in order to achieve a state of deep relaxation.

Counselors also advise better time management. Stress often results from the inability to schedule and prioritize tasks. The pressure of constantly striving to meet material goals can also bring about a case of chronic stress. It is important to treat oneself first before making one's mark on the world. This means pursuing activities not meant to advance a career or result in a specific accomplishment. Simple fun and relaxation is a common prescription for stress. For many people, following this course of *inaction* takes time and practice—in a goal-oriented world, any time out can bring a sense of guilt and time wasted.

Achieving the positive results of stress treatment can take months or years. The key is not to return to old habits.

STRESS MANAGEMENT PROGRAMS

A course of treatment may do little to eliminate the source of stress, making it necessary to follow up with a program of stress management. This combines a change in personal work and living habits, new exercise and diet routines, counseling methods, and certain other techniques designed to strengthen the body's defenses against stress.

The goals of stress management are to change or eliminate the source of stress, if possible; effect a change in attitude that allows a person to better cope with stress; ease the physical effects of stress by taking better care of the body; and learn new ways of dealing with stressful situations when they arise.

A patient in a stress management program learns relaxation techniques such as meditation or Progressive Muscle Relaxation. This kind of treatment is designed to give a person more control over his or her body's or mind's responses to stressful episodes. By becoming more sensitive to one's reactions to stress, an individual can control his or her own anxiety or level of stress. He or she can react quickly and take the most useful steps to reduce the physical and mental wear and tear that will result.

Many alternative methods of treating stress have become popular. These include aromatherapy, the use of relaxing scents; massage and reflexology (foot massage), designed to relieve muscular tension; breathing exercises; yoga sessions; and biofeedback sessions, in which the body's reactions to physical work are shown on gauges or meters.

Q & A

Question: What are people doing to ease their stress?

Answer: According to a 2007 survey, it depends on your gender. The most common approach for women is to talk to their family and friends; 39 percent tried it, while only 19 percent of men tried to relieve stress by talking it out. The next best methods for women were eating more (36 percent) and sleeping more (32 percent). For men, sleeping more and eating more were tied at 25 percent.

Hypnosis

A session of hypnosis can implant a stress-coping mechanism in the unconscious mind. A hypnotist is similar to a coach, who works with the patient in a cooperative way to access the **subconscious** mind. According to one study, however, not everyone is susceptible to hypnosis. The research found that only 15 percent of people are very responsive to hypnosis, and 10 percent are not responsive at all.

In hypnosis, a professional counselor creates a relaxed state known as a hypnotic trance. The person under hypnosis remains aware but also open to suggestions made by the hypnotist. The mind acts on these suggestions without the normal screening process used by the conscious mind. Normal distractions, either from the surroundings or from the subject's own train of thought, are absent.

Those under hypnosis can use suggestions to improve their ability to cope with stress. The suggestion may take the form of a response: "I can deal with this," for example, or "This situation can be fixed." The response arrives from the memory and the subconscious when a stressful situation appears. Posthypnotic suggestions also can help to shape a more positive attitude to settings that have to be faced on a daily basis, such as work or school.

Counseling Methods

Psychotherapy is a form of one-on-one counseling that helps patients to carefully examine their own lives and their view of the world. By talking out their problems and anxieties with a psychiatrist (also a medical doctor) or psychologist, patients can better sort out their priorities and get a grip on stressful situations. Through therapy, they learn to understand why they meet these situations with fear, anxiety, or a strong negative reaction. Patients in therapy learn to better communicate their feelings, to control their anger, and to resolve conflicts with family, friends, or coworkers.

Cognitive therapy allows patients to gain better control of their own emotions and reactions. Many people see themselves as naturally high-strung or energetic, for example, type A personalities who constantly strive for goals and improvement. If a person is suffering symptoms of stress, however, that person's own traits may be driving him or her into self-destructive behaviors, habits, and attitudes. A course of cognitive therapy helps people control their reactions and behavior.

As stress affects a growing number of people and stress management is a growing field of study, many companies offer stress management programs to their employees. These are designed to head off the more serious outcomes of chronic stress and lower the costs of treatment for people suffering illness as a result of their reactions to the pressures of work or study.

Stress management also is evident in high schools across the country, in response to a wave of negative reactions to stress among students. The programs are usually tailored differently for boys and girls. One study in Baltimore found that of all boys experiencing stress, about 48 percent either sought distractions or avoided dealing with it altogether. The figure for girls was much lower—only 33 percent. The study also found that sources of stress were different: For girls, the sources were mainly relationships with boys or conflicts with friends; for boys, conflict came from interaction with authority figures such as teachers, administrators, or coaches. As a result, stress management in schools often means separating girls and boys, emphasizing conflict resolution for boys and one-on-one counseling for girls.

See also: Medication; Meditation; Relaxation Therapies; Stress Management Techniques; Types of Stress

FURTHER READING

Eason, Adam. *The Secrets of Self-Hypnosis: Harnessing the Power of Your Unconscious Mind.* Eagan, Minn.: Network3000 Publishing, 2005.

Rose, Opal. *Dark Water: Stress After Trauma.* Bloomington, Ind.: AuthorHouse, 2007.

Servan-Schreiber, David. *The Instinct to Heal: Curing Stress, Anxiety, and Depression Without Drugs and Without Talk Therapy.* Emmaus, Pa.: Rodale Books, 2004.

■ TYPES OF STRESS

Different psychological and physiological responses to events that upset one's emotional and/or mental balance. Researchers categorize different kinds of stress in different ways. Most of these divisions define either the specific type of stress, its effect on the body, or its intensity and duration.

PHYSICAL STRESS

Physical actions such as running or exercising place the body under physical stress. The heart rate increases, breathing becomes heavy, blood pressure rises, muscles tire, and other symptoms occur from expending the necessary energy to meet the demands placed on the body. Regular physical activity is beneficial to good health, however, and also helps the body deal with periods of mental or emotional stress. Doctors and experts recommend at least 20 minutes of physical activity every day. Such exercise need not be strenuous to improve body functions and overall health. It can be rapid walking, jogging, bicycling, a yoga session, or any team sport that gets the body working.

For some people, vigorous physical exercise can place too much immediate stress on the circulatory system. A body already weakened with heart disease may have an adverse reaction to this kind of stress. The coronary artery can become **ischemic** (starved of sufficient oxygen), resulting in chest pains (angina) or a heart attack.

Physical stress also refers to the effects of any kind of stress on the body's functions. Chronic emotional stress at home, for example, or work-related stress can lead to elevated levels of cortisol and other **stress hormones** in the bloodstream, which can bring high blood pressure, sleeplessness, and other symptoms. Cortisol can have another long-term effect, as one of its important functions is to convert protein and fat into glucose, which is more useful to the body in a short-term emergency. This process, if repeated and chronic, can cause weight loss, hyperglycemia (elevated blood glucose levels), and a feeling of constant fatigue.

In stressed individuals, the **diving reflex** diverts blood from less vital to more important organs. The result, if the stress is chronic, can be cold and clammy skin, ulcers, loss of appetite, digestion problems, and muscular aches and pains. The elevation of blood pressure and the heart rate, as well as the dilation of blood vessels, in repeated stressful episodes can also bring about chest pains, shortness of breath, headaches, heart palpitations, and feelings of alternating chill and fever.

Poor diet, in which needed nutrients are lacking, also stresses the body. Combined with bad eating, chronic stress can affect the body's ability to eliminate cholesterol, which can build up in the arteries that pump blood to the heart. It also affects the immune system and can worsen certain health conditions such as allergies, skin conditions, and asthma.

Psychological Effects

A body subjected to frequent stress will begin to show psychological as well as physical symptoms, caused by elevated levels of stress hormones such as cortisol and their by-products, such as glucose. This is the reason for the many mental symptoms of a chronically stressed person: anxiety, depression, mood swings, irritability, an inability to concentrate, and the greater likelihood of addiction to alcohol or narcotics.

EMOTIONAL STRESS

A common form of stress is emotional stress brought about by confrontation, the pressure of work, family troubles, constant anxiety, or grieving. Emotional stress produces a state of tension in which the mind focuses on the problem at hand to the exclusion of everything else. Thoughts race out of control, with the mind attempting to resolve difficult situations and strained relationships. Emotional stress can cause restlessness and a sense of panic when a person feels he or she is losing control of events. It can drastically affect performance at work or school, making it impossible to concentrate, meet the expectations of a boss, or solve a problem.

Outer signs of emotional stress include angry outbursts and irritation at minor problems such as losing a pair of gloves or the appearance of rain that slows traffic. People under emotional stress can appear nervous and shy, sometimes fearful in the presence of strangers. They tend to withdraw from the world and may not be responsive to questions, comments, or any attempt at conversation.

Fact Or Fiction?

Stress turns your hair gray.

The Facts: Overproduction of stress hormones interferes with the production of melanin, a pigmenting agent used by hair follicles to impart color to the hair. Research studies have shown that people under higher amounts of chronic stress tend to have more gray hair than their relatively unstressed peers.

MENTAL STRESS

Mental stress is an effect of physical or emotional stress, which can disrupt the ability to work through problems using mental calculation, logic, and memory. People undergoing a stressful event such as a sudden emergency or a car accident find themselves unable to think or carry out normal mental processes. They may be unable to concentrate or even speak properly; they may act in a disjointed or illogical manner. In an attempt to regain their thinking ability, they may concentrate intensely on a simple action, one that they would normally carry out without thinking at all. They also may have periods of amnesia, when the memory of a person or event is lost.

Chronic mental stress can lead to behavior that further stresses the physical body. This includes smoking, heavy alcohol use, and unhealthy eating. Of course, different people have different mental responses to stress. Some welcome a certain amount of pressure and uncertainty in their lives, and they cope with that stress better than others. As long as one is engaged with others, a completely stressless life is impossible to achieve. Human interaction gives rise to stress, but this interaction is also necessary, to a certain extent, for mental balance and happiness.

Fact Or Fiction?

Smoking relieves stress.

The Facts: Smokers will often turn to a cigarette for relief from a stressful situation. They may do this to escape or to gain a temporary feeling of relief from the release of endorphins that smoking brings about. However, smoking to deal with stress is not a very good idea. As a stimulant, nicotine (the active ingredient in cigarette smoke) actually creates an elevated stress level. People who smoke suffer more from stress than nonsmokers, and their general level of health is not as good as nonsmokers. In fact, smoking places more stress on the body than it relieves.

ACUTE STRESS

Researchers also classify stress in terms of duration and intensity. Acute stress happens suddenly in response to a threat or emergency. It can result from a real or imaginary problem. It happens when a person is startled or suddenly made aware of danger.

Whether the danger is real or just imagined, a bout of acute stress triggers a response in the autonomic nervous system. On a signal from the pituitary gland and hypothalamus in the brain, the **endocrine system** releases a wave of stress hormones into the bloodstream through the adrenal glands, which rest atop the kidneys. Blood is diverted from the skin and extremities to the major muscle groups and the vital organs, the heart rate increases, and the body prepares to fight or run away.

The stressful episode eventually passes or is resolved, and the stress response subsides. In the process of **homeostasis,** the body's self-regulating system returns levels of hormones in the bloodstream, as well as physical responses, to normal.

Some individuals seek out episodes of acute stress. Attracted to danger and the rush of **adrenaline,** they take up skydiving, bungee jumping, downhill skiing, or other activities that can bring physical danger. The body's ability to cope with such activities is limited, however, and repeated acute stress can bring a sense of fatigue and anxiety, as well as unwanted physical symptoms: headaches, upset stomach, muscle tension.

Other people face episodes of acute stress repeatedly, as a product of their own psychological makeup or their work and life situation. The aggressive, ambitious type A personality places intense demands on him- or herself and others, and as a result suffers a lack of time in which to accomplish goals. Frequent stressful episodes bring about anxiety, irritability, impatience, and depressive episodes. The victim of frequent acute stress also suffers physical effects such as frequent headaches and sleeplessness, as well as a strong sense of insecurity.

CHRONIC STRESS

Not all stress subsides, and when an acute stress episode becomes a repeated experience, the body and mind begin to suffer the symptoms of chronic stress. One way to think of the difference between acute and chronic stress is in terms of time: If a person is asked to write down the causes of stress, he or she will be able to write down only chronic **stressors** (an *acute* stressor would not allow the time to write).

Many people, young and old, are suffering with the problem of chronic stress, as many are experiencing the constant demands of work, or school, or more personal burdens such as marital problems, financial difficulty, and worry about the future. The management of one's time and responsibilities can easily lead to a case of chronic stress. Type A workers, for example, tend to overextend themselves on the job or in school, taking on more responsibilities than they can capably handle in a given amount of time. Although type A personalities are said to "thrive on stress," their work style can easily bring about an unhealthy case of chronic stress, which can in turn affect their ability to function and perform.

Other sources of chronic stress include poor diet, in which the body does not get the nutrients it needs (this is the oldest kind of stress, growing out of the most serious cause of chronic stress for ancient humans: hunger). Chronic stress also can be brought on by a serious illness such as arthritis or a back injury, which causes constant pain. An unhappy marriage, a boring job, failing grades, chaotic finances, and poor health can all bring on chronic stress.

In evolutionary terms, the human system has largely outgrown the need for a "fight-or-flight" response. The stress response was necessary when confronted with immediate physical danger. Most instances of acute stress were soon resolved, one way or another, either by death or by escape and survival. Today, the human stress response survives, preparing us for physical action that, in most cases, is not necessary. The endocrine system that evolved to produce stress hormones is out of step with social and cultural evolution and modern society. For people today, deadly confrontations with wild animals or even human enemies are rarely a problem.

Chronic, low-level stress has serious long-term consequences, however, including an effect on the heart, circulatory system, immune system, and one's mental capacity. Chronic worriers overstimulate their **sympathetic nervous system,** which initiates the stress response, and suppress their **parasympathetic nervous system,** which repairs any damage done by stress hormones and returns the body to its relaxed state. As a result, their heart rates and blood pressure remain too high, their digestion is poor, they feel tired, their sex drive is impaired, and their immune system is compromised, leaving them vulnerable to heart disease, ulcers, and cancer.

EUSTRESS—THE GOOD KIND OF STRESS

Researchers also have identified the concept of eustress, or positive stress, which is beneficial to the functioning of the mind and body. Physical exercise is one form of eustress. Another is a challenging job that engages the mind and demands creativity and some form of problem solving. Eustress helps a person to engage with the world and surrounding people. It keeps the mind focused.

Eustress also comes in the form of hobbies, extracurricular activities, outside interests, and social contacts that require a certain amount of time management and problem-solving ability. Those who miss these aspects of a healthy life may have serious problems coping with

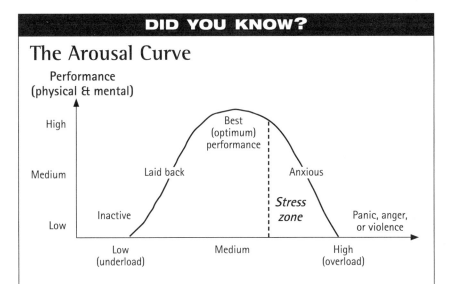

DID YOU KNOW?

The Arousal Curve

Researchers use the "arousal curve" to explain the effect of acute stress and the relationship between arousal and performance. While a medium arousal level contributes to peak performance, in the "stress zone," performance deteriorates as arousal and stress begin to overload the system.

Source: "Fear and Violence in Stressed Populations," at http://www.eoslifework.co.uk/gturmap.htm

acute or chronic stress, as they lack outlets for the mental energy and anxiety they experience. Escape to a familiar, quiet home is a good way to cope with stress, but chronic antisocial behavior gives rise to its own set of mental and physical problems. Along with the stress response, humans have evolved the ability to draw on support networks of familiar people—friends and family—to help them survive life's dangers and uncertainties.

See also: Anniversary Reactions; Emotional Stress; Grieving and Mourning; Stress and the Family; Stress Rating Scales

FURTHER READING
Lovallo, William R. *Stress and Health: Biological and Psychological Interactions*. Thousand Oaks, Calif.: Sage Publications, 2004.

McEwan, Bruce, and Elizabeth Norton Lasley. *The End of Stress as We Know It*. Washington, D.C.: The National Academies, 2004.

Sapolsky, Robert M. *Why Zebras Don't Get Ulcers: The Acclaimed Guide to Stress, Stress-Related Diseases, and Coping*. New York: Henry Holt, 2004.

■ WORKPLACE STRESS

Reactions to conflict on the job and probably the most common form of stress. Although industrialized societies have banished the constant, life-threatening dangers of the past, stress has survived in the workforce with the need for gainful employment, the desire to earn money, and the responsibility of supporting oneself or one's family.

The pressure to earn money and the constantly changing nature of the modern workplace place new forms of emotional stress on the human nervous system. Many jobs result in stress symptoms that are difficult to face if a workplace situation remains the same. The difficulty of finding new employment makes change impossible for many.

The results of workplace stress can be emotional as well as physical. Heart disease, ulcers, high blood pressure, insomnia, anxiety, depression, and breakdowns in the immune system are frequent effects of a stressful job. Burnout is common to many professions, situations in which people have little variety in their tasks and few tasks are designed to engage their interests or challenge their abilities.

Nevertheless, many jobs are fulfilling and provide workers with periods of beneficial eustress, a physical or mental challenge that creates a positive form of stress. Those who report satisfaction with their jobs often see the stressful moments and challenges as the best part of their employment. Without such challenges, a daily routine repeated for years can bring a heavy sense of boredom and frustration, two of the most common factors in a worker's report of stress on the job.

TYPES A AND B

The experience of stress on the job varies with the individual. Psychologists have classified workers and employers with two basic personality types, A and B. The type A personality tends to thrive on stress, seeks out tough assignments, often provokes confrontations, feels a keen sense of competition with others, easily grows impatient, and may be hungry for attention and praise. Type A individuals typically overschedule themselves, trying to do two or more things at once and to accomplish more than can be reasonably expected in a working day. They tend to speak quickly, interrupt more frequently, and may easily become suspicious, hostile, and angry.

Type B individuals tend to seek contentment through cooperation with others, avoid confrontations, and feel less pressure for the boss's praise and recognition. Type B people pay less attention to the clock and the necessity of finishing an assignment on time. Although they are slow to anger, they are more prone to boredom and tend to lack motivation.

"Adrenaline Junkies"

According to many researchers, there is an important physical difference between types A and B: a higher level of **stress hormones** in type A individuals, which brings about their more intense reaction to challenges in the workplace. As a result of elevated stress hormone levels, type A individuals might also be more prone to high blood pressure, headaches, and heart attacks.

Type B individuals, with lower stress hormone levels, react quite differently to mental and physical **stressors**. As a result of lower average stress hormones in their system, they might be better equipped to handle workplace stress without physical damage.

The stress hormones **cortisol** and **adrenaline** may take a longer time to "wash out" from a type A individual, which would be a key reason for sleeplessness at night and a feeling of constant fatigue during the day. There are many driven individuals who thrive on stress and stress hormones, however, and who purposely seek out situations they know will bring the stress reaction. These "adrenaline junkies" can be found in dangerous occupations, among police officers, firefighters, deep-sea fishers, military pilots, and the most hazardous job of all: logging (who die at the rate of almost 118 per 100,000 workers, the highest rate of workplace fatalities in the United States). Stress is a key component of these occupations and an important reason why people active in these professions tend to have shorter careers and take an earlier retirement. Simply the prospect of facing a potentially dangerous situation often provides the type A person with a form of job fulfillment.

Men and Women
Researchers have also found that the stress of the workplace has different effects on men and women. While a man might react to and relieve stress with anger, expressed outward, a stressed women is more likely to keep anger and hostility to herself and may grow polite, silent, and distant when under pressure from superiors. Women also have difficulty setting priorities between a demanding family and a difficult work situation, both of which may be sources of conflict. While a man under pressure may choose to neglect the needs of children, the home, or a marriage, women may feel less inclined to turn away from the home situation and consequently feel a keen sense of guilt and responsibility. In fact, the rate of stress-related illnesses is growing faster among women than among men, who in many societies have culturally more acceptable physical outlets for that stress than women do.

Q & A

Question: Isn't there a law about workplace stress?

Answer: There are many federal and state laws controlling work environments and the employer/employee relationship. The Occupational Safety and Health Administration (OSHA) regulates workplace safety. The Equal Employment Opportunity Commission (EEOC) deals with workplace discrimination and harassment. It is a civil rights violation to discriminate against anyone in the workplace based on his or her age, race, gender, political beliefs, disability, sexual orientation, or religious affiliation. It is also against the law to create a hostile work environment for employees. However, simply creating "stress" for a worker—caused by the amount or type of work to be done—is not grounds for a lawsuit.

WORK STRESSORS

Physical danger, of course, is not the only source of workplace stress. Those workers who bear responsibility for the safety of others experience high stress. This includes firefighters, hospital workers, paramedics, and air-traffic controllers; ironically, a high percentage of people with stressful jobs report feeling a sense of job satisfaction—which arises from how certain personality types also match certain occupations.

In a job without physical dangers, a wide range of psychological and emotional stressors may be present as a consequence of the boss, the coworkers, the work itself, or a worker who may have taken employment that simply was not suited to his or her personality. Demanding bosses will exert pressure to make deadlines, fulfill sales quotas, or handle a large volume of requests from clients and customers. Colleagues at work might strive to outdo one another in production, undercut the efforts of rivals, curry favor with managers, or sabotage the efforts of coworkers, all in an effort to get ahead. Office politics—the entire range of social behaviors present in a working environment among coworkers—can provide a constant source of anxiety and emotional stress.

The most intense and damaging form of stress in a workplace comes from a sense of powerlessness. Workers who have little control over how much work they do, or how they do their jobs, feel employed at the whim of others (or, frequently, the whims of the ever-changing demands of a commercial market). Many factory workers, assemblers, and textile workers must carry out tasks that simply do not challenge their real abilities. They are offered fewer rewards and recognition, and with less responsibility or technical ability comes mediocre pay. In such situations, periods of high stress are common. Anyone carrying out a repetitive task, and who has little prospect of changing jobs or routines, experiences more stress than normal and is the most likely to experience job burnout.

Another factor in workplace stress is schedule. Those who work night shifts live in conflict with the natural circadian rhythm of their bodies, which seek sleep at the coming of darkness. Those with irregular schedules or who work short intense periods followed by a long break also experience higher levels of stress. Frequent travel and public contact add to workplace stress.

COPING WITH WORKPLACE STRESS

Psychologists have generally concluded that changing the basic work personality of an individual is not possible or even desirable. Also, there are deep-seated social factors at work. Type A individuals, for example, in the United States and other countries, are generally admired for their ambition, goal orientation, energy, commitment, and achievements.

Instead of "curing" the type, the potentially damaging aspects of a type A or type B personality can be addressed: A tendency to hostile outbreaks in a type A, for example, can be handled with a course in anger management; type B individuals can be motivated with a wider range of responsibilities and a more varied work schedule. There are a variety of other strategies available to workers of either type to help deal with stress on the job.

Communication

Workers experiencing stress should communicate their situation to their employer and try to work out a solution. In some cases, a change of schedule or new assignment can help someone deal with a case of job burnout. A manager seeking to avoid burnout in employees should train workers thoroughly, communicate expectations clearly, and try to offer some reward or verbal recognition for work done satisfactorily.

Time Management

To avoid negative reactions to stressors, workers should avoid over-scheduling themselves and committing to more work than they can accomplish. In turn, when an assignment is undertaken, they should carefully plan to finish the work with a planner or calendar.

Rest and Recovery

Jobs that place a lot of demands on workers should also offer regular work breaks. Workers seeking to avoid stress should give themselves a block of downtime during the day—during a lunch break, for example—to escape the scene or turn to an enjoyable physical or mental activity.

If possible, work also should be avoided away from the workplace. Anyone working a job that demands long hours at the office should allow themselves time at home during which they have an opportu-

DID YOU KNOW?

The Most and Least Stressful Jobs in America

Most Stressful Jobs

1. Surgeon
2. Commercial pilot
3. Photojournalist
4. Advertising account executive
5. Real estate agent
6. Physician
7. Newspaper reporter
8. Physician's assistant

Least Stressful Jobs

1. Actuary (compiles statistics for insurance companies)
2. Dietitian
3. Computer analyst
4. Statistician
5. Astronomer
6. Mathematician
7. Historian
8. Software engineer

The report lists the country's most stressful and least stressful jobs.

Source: "2009 Jobs Rated Report," Careercast.com.

nity to temporarily forget their job duties. This also is true for vacation and holiday time.

Life in Balance

Another key weapon in the fight against stress is to maintain an active social life and interact with friends and acquaintances as often as possible. In many studies, researchers have found that people who tend to isolate themselves from others are more prone to the physical damages of stress. A stressed worker can balance the demands of a job with time for hobbies and exercise, providing enough time for sleep at night, keeping to a healthy diet, and striving to keep an optimistic outlook. Often a negative and pessimistic attitude contributes as much to stress as the work situation itself. Avoiding heavy self-criticism and negative vocabulary such as *impossible* and *never* in the inner dialogue will eventually result in a sense of self-worth and optimism.

Stress Management Techniques

Common stress management techniques are useful in combating pressures at work. These include daily sessions of meditation or yoga, a regular exercise routine, autogenic training, Progressive Muscle Relaxation, or biofeedback sessions. All can be undertaken either alone or with the guidance of an instructor. Any therapy that allows the mind to focus inward and temporarily clear out work and its worries can help to alleviate reactions to stress.

See also: Performance Anxiety; Stress and the Environment; Types of Stress

FURTHER READING

Culbert, Samuel. *Beyond Bullsh*t: Straight-Talk at Work.* Stanford, Calif.: Stanford Business Publications, 2008.

King, Melanie. *Surviving Stress at Work: Understand It, Overcome It.* Bloomington, Ind.: Trafford Publishing, 2006.

Leiter, Michael P. *Banishing Burnout: Six Strategies for Improving Your Relationship with Work.* San Francisco: Jossey-Bass, 2005.

HOTLINES AND HELP SITES

Active Minds
URL: www.activemindsoncampus.org
Phone: 1-202-332-9595
Mission: Peer-to-peer organization dedicated to raising awareness about mental health among college students
Programs: The young adult voice in mental health advocacy on more than 100 college campuses nationwide

Anxiety Disorders Association of America
URL: www.adaa.org
Phone: 1-240-485-1001
Address: 11900 Parklawn Drive, Suite 100 Rockville, MD 20852-2624
Mission: To promote the prevention, treatment, and cure of anxiety disorders and to improve the lives of people who suffer from them

Crisis Link
URL: http://www.crisislink.org
Phone: 1-800-273-8255
Mission: To provide support to those facing life crises, traumas, and suicide
Programs: 24/7 Crisis & Suicide Prevention Hotlines; CareRing phone check-in for the elderly and disabled; You Talk, We Listen targeted suicide and crisis prevention outreach to youth; Crisis Response Team; Community Education

International Critical Incident Stress Management Team
Coordination Center
URL: http://www.icisf.org/hotline.htm
Phone: 410-313-2473
Mission: To assist responders with the traumatic stress they often
encounter when dealing with accidents, fires, hostage situations,
and other emergencies
Programs: Coordinates a network of 400 Critical Incident Stress
Management (CISM) teams throughout all 50 states and 16 foreign
countries and maintains a 24-hour hotline

National Institute of Mental Health
URL: http://www.nimh.nih.gov/
Phone: 1-301-443-4513
Mission: To reduce the burden of mental illness and behavioral disorders through research on the mind, brain, and behavior
Programs: Support the science of brain and behavior as a foundation
for understanding mental disorders; define genetic and environmental risk factors; develop safe, effective, equitable treatments;
support clinical trials; rapidly disseminate science information to
mental health-care professionals and services

Parent Hotline
URL: http://parenthotline.net
Phone: 1-800-840-6537
Mission: Parent Hotline works with schools and programs across the
country to assist parents and families with a struggling teen
Programs: Facilitates the enrollment of students in specialty and
boarding schools in several locations

Stress Management Support Group
URL: http://www.dailystrength.org/c/Stress-Management/support-
group
Mission: Provides a large network of support groups for people facing
physical, emotional, and psychological challenges
Programs: Ask an Expert feature allows users to pose questions
directly to health professionals

TeenLine

URL: www.teenlineonline.org

Phone: 310-855-HOPE

       800-TLC-TEEN

Address: P.O. Box 48750

Los Angeles, CA 90048

Mission: To assist teenagers in trouble or with questions through an evening help line, e-mail, online chat, and message boards. Volunteers are teenagers trained to clarify concerns, give options, and help callers positive decisions

Programs: Teen Suicide Prevention Workshop; Teen Suicide Prevention Training for Law Enforcement; Teen Line Outreach for At-Risk Youth; Teen Line/Sheldon Andelson LGBT Outreach; Drug & Alcohol Abuse Prevention Outreach

GLOSSARY

acute   sudden onset or short term

addiction   a chronic, relapsing condition or disease characterized by compulsive   alcohol, tobacco, or drug seeking and abuse and by long-lasting chemical changes in the brain

adrenal gland   controls the body's autonomic nervous system

adrenaline   a hormone secreted in the adrenal gland and produced in response to fear

aerobic exercise   vigorous, repetitive exercise such as walking, running, or swimming that increases breathing, raises the heart rate, and uses up oxygen in your blood

agoraphobia   severe anxiety about being in open or public areas; literally means "a fear of the marketplace"

alprazolam   a tranquilizer; brand name *Xanax*

amitriptyline   an antidepressant occurring as a white or nearly white crystalline powder, administered orally or intramuscularly

amoxapine   an antidepressant

amygdala   one of the basal ganglia: a roughly almond-shaped mass of gray matter deep inside each cerebral hemisphere

anniversary stress physical and psychological reactions to prior traumatic events, with the reactions occurring on a yearly basis after the event

anxiety disorder abnormal sense of fear, doubt about reality of the source of the fear, and self-doubt about coping with it

arrhythmia any variation from the normal rhythm of the heart beat

attention deficit disorder most common neurobiological behavioral disorder in children; symptoms include distractibility and impulsivity

autonomic nervous system the part of the nervous system that controls involuntary body actions such as the beating of the heart

benzodiazepines drugs used to treat anxiety, as well as seizures and delirium associated with alcohol withdrawal syndrome

beta-blockers fast-acting and nonhabit-forming drugs used to calm anxiety symptoms such as shaking, palpitations, and excessive perspiration

binge eating a mental condition in which a person periodically consumes huge amounts of food in a short period of time

bupropion an antidepressant medication that works by enhancing the release of dopamine and **norepinephrine;** used when side effects such as weight gain and drowsiness need to be avoided

chlordiazepoxide a sedative used for the treatment of mild anxiety and the reduction of nervous and muscular tension

chronic used to describe any illness such as alcoholism that is not easily cured

chronic stress a state of elevated physical or emotional stress that continues for a lengthy period of time and which can eventually result in higher blood pressure and other adverse health effects

citalopram   an antidepressant and antianxiety drug sold under the brand names of Celexa and Cipramil; belonging to the family of **selective serotonin reuptake inhibitors (SSRIs)**

clonazepam   a medication used for the treatment of anxiety, panic disorder, and seizure disorders

corticotropin   a hormone secreted by the pituitary gland in response to stress, and which prompts the release of stress hormone **cortisol** into the bloodstream

corticotropin-releasing factor   a chemical produced by the **hypothalamus,** and which regulates the body's response to stress, anxiety, and depression

cortisol   a hormone produced by the body when under stress

depression   a mental condition characterized by feelings of extreme sadness or worthlessness, loss of interest in pleasurable activities, changes in sleep or appetite patterns, fatigue, and difficulty in concentrating

desipramine   an antidepressant medication that is used in the treatment of depression, drug withdrawal, and attention deficit disorder

diazepam   a popular medication developed in the 1960s, sold under the brand name Valium, and used for the treatment of anxiety, depression, muscle spasms, insomnia, and symptoms of alcoholism

distress   the inability to adapt to the presence of stress and the resulting physical and emotional symptoms such as withdrawal, depression, and aggression

diving reflex   the body's reaction to contact with water, in which the heart slows, blood vessels constrict, and blood circulation to the muscles and abdomen decreases

doxepin   a medication used in the treatment of insomnia, anxiety, and depression; sold under the brand names Aponal, Deptran, and Adapine

duloxetine a medication used in the treatment of depression and anxiety; sold under the brand name Cymbalta

endocrine   system the system of ductless glands that regulate bodily functions through hormones secreted into the bloodstream

endorphins natural substances produced by the pituitary gland and **hypothalamus** that regulates a variety of things, including reducing pain, hunger, and the release of sex hormones

enkephalins peptide **neurotransmitters** that help control the body's psychological response to pain

escitalopram an antidepressant medication sold under the brand names Lexapro and Cipralex

eustress "good stress" with the quality of enhancing mood and helping the individual function normally and cope with the demands of home and/or work

"fight-or-flight" response a physical reaction that prepares the human body for extreme activity; the body's automatic and involuntary reaction to a frightening situation

fluoxetine an antidepressant medication used for depression and panic disorder; sold under the brand name Prozac

fluvoxamine an antidepressant medication used to treat anxiety disorders, obsessive compulsive disorder, and **post-traumatic stress disorder**; currently sold under the brand name Luvox

glucocorticoids naturally occurring hormones that control the production of glucose and also regulate the response of the **immune system**

glucogen a hormone that controls the level of blood sugar in the body, raising blood sugar when levels decrease, enhancing energy

guided imagery a technique in which an individual is instructed to imagine a series of scenes and various sensory stimuli that help to reduce stress levels

homeostasis the body's process of maintaining equilibrium; for example, eating because one's energy level is low

hormones a chemical substance that some cells in the body release to help other cells work; for example, insulin is a hormone that helps the body use glucose as energy

hyperstress a period of elevated stress in which an individual loses control of his or her physical or emotional reaction to the **stressor**

hypertension constant elevated blood pressure levels, which can damage the heart and arteries and which, in the opinion of some researchers, can lead to coronary artery disease and heart attack

hypostress a period of little or no stress or challenge that can bring about boredom and restlessness

hypothalamus region of the brain that regulates certain body functions, including water balance, temperature, and the production of the hormones in the pituitary gland

imipramine an antidepressant medication used for panic disorder and depression; sold under the brand names Deprimin, Deprinol, and others

immune system the cells and organs in the body that fight disease and infection

ischemic tending to cause a constriction in blood vessels and blood circulation to the extremities, or to the brain, heart, or other organs

isocaboxazid an antidepressant medication that is **toxic** to the body and has generally fallen out of use

lorazepam a medication used for treatment of anxiety, seizures, and insomnia, and as a sedative

maprotiline a medication used for treatment of anxiety, panic attacks, and depression

mirtazapine an antidepressant medication sold under the brand names Remeron, Avanza, and Zispin

neurotransmitters   a neurochemical such as serotonin that attaches to a receptor in the brain to transfer signals between a neuron and another cell

norepenephrine   a hormone and a **neurotransmitter** secreted by the adrenal glands that governs the body's **autonomic nervous system,** especially blood pressure and heart rate; prepares the body for stress

nortriptyline   a medication used to treat depression, chronic fatigue, and migraine headaches; sold under the brand name Sensoval and others

oxytocin   a hormone that is secreted by the pituitary gland and that plays an important role in sexual reproduction, pregnancy, and birth by reducing anxiety

parasympathetic nervous system   the area of the nervous system that calms the body; works with the **sympathetic nervous system** (SNS)

paroxetine   a medication, one of the **selective serotonin reuptake inhibitors** (SSRIs); used to treat depression and anxiety and sold under the brand name Paxil

phenelzine   an antidepressant and antianxiety medication sold under the brand name Nardil

pituitary   (gland) a small oval endocrine gland that lies at the base of the brain; sometimes called the master gland because all of the other endocrine glands depend on its secretion for stimulation

placebo   a pill containing no medication; administered for its psychological effect in medical studies

postholiday financial stress syndrome   a condition of heightened stress and anxiety brought on by money worries after the holiday gift-giving season has concluded

post-traumatic stress disorder   an anxiety disorder characterized by a severe and recurring emotional reaction to a traumatic event such as a violent assault or war

prefrontal cortex   a region of the frontal lobes of the brain that regulates social interaction, planning, and the expression of individual personality

prolactin   a hormone secreted by the pituitary gland that helps to regulate the flow of breast milk during lactation

protriptyline   an antidepressant that is sold under the brand name Vivactil; is also used to treat chronic pain

selective serotonin reuptake inhibitors   ·an antidepressant that acts on the chemical in the brain called **serotonin** and is used in the treatment of depression, anxiety disorders, and some personality disorders

selegiline   a medication that is used to combat depression and which is known for its ability to combat the symptoms of Parkinson's disease

self-esteem   the sense of value one attributes to oneself

serotonin   a **neurotransmitter** or chemical that inhibits self-destructive behavior; also affects a person's mood and feelings of being hungry or full

serotonin syndrome   a condition brought on by an excessive release of **serotonin,** usually caused by a drug reaction, and causing nausea, restlessness, hallucinations, changes in blood pressure, vomiting, and diarrhea

sertraline   an antidepressant medication sold under the brand name Zoloft

sibling rivalry   competition between brothers and sisters for their parents' attention, approval, and protection

sphygmomanometer   a device that measures blood pressure, using an inflatable cuff placed around the arm and a scaled meter to measure pressure

stress hormones   chemicals, including **cortisol** and **norepinephrine,** that are released into the bloodstream at periods of physical or emotional stress and that cause reactions that prepare the body for "fight or flight"

stressor a factor or event that precipitates or drives a negative behavior or outcome

subconscious part of the mind below the level of awareness

sympathetic nervous system the area of the nervous system that revs up the body's system; balances the **parasympathetic nervous system** (PNS), which later calms the body

toxic poisonous

tranylcypromine a medication used to treat depression and anxiety; sold under the brand name Parnate

trimipramine a medication used to treat depression, insomnia, alcoholism, and chronic pain; sold under the brand name Surmontil

vasopressin a hormone that is released from the pituitary gland and that has several functions, including water retention, control of blood pressure, and various brain functions, including memory and sleep rhythms

venlafaxine an antidepressant medication used for the treatment of panic disorder and anxiety; marketed as Effexor or Efexor

INDEX

Page numbers in *italic* indicate graphs or sidebars. **Boldface** page numbers indicate extensive treatment of a topic.